THE ATHLETIC BRAIN

THE ATHLETIC BRAIN

How Neuroscience Is Revolutionising Sport and Can Help You Perform Better

AMIT KATWALA

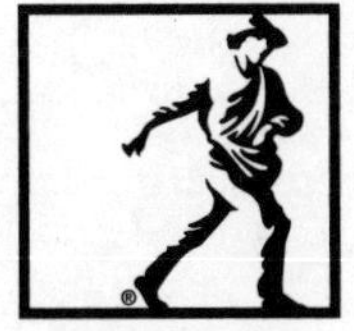

SIMON & SCHUSTER

London · New York · Sydney · Toronto · New Delhi

A CBS COMPANY

First published in Great Britain by Simon & Schuster UK Ltd, 2016
A CBS COMPANY

1 3 5 7 9 10 8 6 4 2

Simon & Schuster UK Ltd
1st Floor
222 Gray's Inn Road
London WC1X 8HB

www.simonandschuster.co.uk

Simon & Schuster Australia, Sydney
Simon & Schuster India, New Delhi

A CIP catalogue record for this book
is available from the British Library.

ISBN: 978-1-4711-5590-1
Trade paperback ISBN: 978-1-4711-5649-6
Ebook ISBN: 978-1-4711-5592-5

Typeset in Minion by M Rules
Printed and bound by CPI Group (UK) Ltd, Croydon, CR0 4YY

Simon & Schuster UK Ltd are committed to sourcing paper
that is made from wood grown in sustainable forests and support the Forest
Stewardship Council, the leading international forest certification organisation.
Our books displaying the FSC logo are printed on FSC certified paper.

To my parents, for a home full of books

And to Sara, for building one with me

"Behind every action there must be a thought"

– Dennis Bergkamp

CONTENTS

INTRODUCTION

Wayne Rooney is lying unconscious on the kitchen floor. In March 2015, footage emerged online of the England and Manchester United striker appearing to be knocked out in a light-hearted boxing match with a friend in his Cheshire home. It wasn't the first time Rooney's head has made headlines. There are stories about whether it's in the right place whenever his form drops, and there were plenty of puzzled takes on the hair transplant he revealed in June 2011.

But few reports paused to acknowledge the role played by Rooney's head in one of the biggest *on*-pitch stories of his career. On 12 February 2011, he scored the winner in a tight 2-1 win over Manchester City which played a vital role in securing United's 19th top-flight English title. Late in the game, a deflected cross from the right-hand side looped up, just behind where Rooney was waiting in the area. He turned and, with his back to goal, elected to try the audacious – launching himself into the air to pull off a stunning overhead kick into the top corner.

In 2012, it was voted the greatest goal in the first 20 years of the Premier League, with over a quarter of the vote. The goal was a triumph of quick thinking and improvisation – a goal that owed as much to Rooney's brain as it did to his body. 'When a cross comes into the box, there are so many things that go through your mind in a split second, like five or six different things you can do with the ball,'

Rooney told *ESPN* magazine, when asked to describe the decision-making process that led him to opt for the out-of-this-world.

'You're asking yourself six questions in a split second. Maybe you've got time to bring it down on the chest and shoot, or you have to head it first time. If the defender is there, you've obviously got to hit it first time. If he's farther back, you've got space to take a touch. You get the decision made. Then it's obviously about the execution.'

This is a book about decision-making.

Rooney isn't the quickest or the tallest – he's relatively short, stocky and has frequently been accused of carrying too much weight. He left school at 16 with no qualifications, as the tongue-in-cheek tattoo on his arm that references the Stereophonics' album *Just Enough Education to Perform* attests to. However, Rooney's mind is active, sharp and agile; this is what gives him the edge over those who might be more physically capable.

Rooney did get an education – on patches of grass on the council estate in Croxteth, Liverpool, where he grew up, despite the signs prohibiting ball games, and in his grandmother's back garden, despite her frustration at him ruining the pebbledash walls. All that experience changed him and made him the player he is today.

As much as their muscles, it is their incredibly specialised brains that make elite athletes different. The differences may not be as easy to spot as the chunky thigh muscles of sprint cyclists or the cauliflower ears of rugby players, but look closely enough and they are there.

This is a book about how practice changes the brain.

In *Outliers*, Malcolm Gladwell popularised the '10,000-hour rule' – the idea that it takes 10,000 hours of deliberate practice to become an expert in any field, including sport. Spectacular goals don't come from nowhere. They are the result of years of practice and hard work. Rooney first came on to Manchester United's radar playing against them at under-9s level, a 12-2 Everton win in which he scored six goals. 'There was one goal that stood out,' remembered Paul McGuinness, who was coaching the United side that day. 'It was basically the classic overhead kick, the perfect bicycle kick, which for a kid of eight or nine years old was really something special.'

Rooney has supplemented all that physical practice by training his brain. Before every game, he visualises himself performing well against the upcoming opponents. 'I lie in bed the night before the game and visualise myself scoring goals or doing well,' he has said. 'You're trying to put yourself in that moment and trying to prepare yourself, to have a "memory" before the game. I don't know if you'd call it visualising or dreaming, but I've always done it, my whole life.'

He's not alone. Psychologists and neuroscientists are unlocking the secrets of the athletic brain, and using that knowledge to develop new training tools that can help amateurs become better, and push elite athletes to new peaks of performance.

This is a book about breaking the 10,000-hour rule.

It's about why athletes choke and how to stop them. It's about scouting for innate sporting talent and decision-making under pressure. It's about pushing the limits of endurance, hacking our way into the zone, and revealing the damage caused by sporting concussions. It's about finding out what makes the best athletes different, and then figuring out how to close the gap.

This is a book about unleashing the endless potential of the human brain, and changing sport forever.

But it starts with a clumsy robot on a crooked pitch.

Part One

THE ATHLETIC BRAIN

CHAPTER ONE

CRISTIANO RONALDO AND THE ART OF ANTICIPATION

In a sweltering arena on the north-east coast of Brazil, the competition is heating up. It's the summer of 2014. The English team's star striker races down the left, arcs his run to open up an angle for the shot . . . and scuffs it horribly. In fact, it's such a bad effort that the ball starts to roll backwards on the uneven pitch, away from the goal, to anguished shouts from the crowd. Undeterred, the tireless forward turns as his software calculates a new course towards the ball. His motors whir in pursuit, but it's too late. The final whistle sounds, and England's hopes are extinguished.

It's the World Cup, but not as you know it.

The English striker in this game doesn't bear much resemblance to your usual international footballer, although he has clocked up similar mileage travelling around the world to competitions. Mustachio is not very good in the air, his first touch isn't great, and he's wearing a miniature top hat and a monocle. He is a 40-centimetre (16-inch) tall 'humanoid robot', part of the University of Plymouth team competing at the 2014 RoboCup.

He does have a bit more in common with the likes of Wayne Rooney than it seems at first glance. The robot's software is designed to tackle the same problems that Rooney's brain has to handle when he is on the pitch. It's designed to use similar strategies, starting with working out where the ball is, and where it's going to be next.

Mustachio, and his Plymouth teammates Pixel, Gears, Amps and Flux, use identical webcams to collect the visual information they need. Like humans, they can then use that data to work out the trajectory and path of the ball, and make decisions based on its movements. Despite the high technology on display, the game is excruciatingly slow. That's mainly down to the lumbering gait of the robots, though – a major stumbling block according to Dr Phil Culverhouse, one of Mustachio's creators. He seems genuinely delighted as he reports that none of Plymouth's players fell over during the competition in Brazil.

Sport is a deceptively difficult thing for the brain to do. The simplest of movements requires precise calculations of the speed and trajectory of objects, and of our own position in space. 'There is more computational power in picking up a chess piece and moving it than there is in deciding the chess move,' says Dr Vincent Walsh of University College London, one of the world's leading cognitive neuroscientists. 'I don't think sport gets the respect it deserves in terms of brain processing power. It is a form of intelligence.'

That's why the robots remain so far behind. Our brains are still much quicker and more complex. 'The human system is incredibly complicated,' says Culverhouse, from his office at Plymouth's Centre for Robotics and Neural Science. 'Humans have the benefit of some absolutely amazing real-time processing going on in the brain, so we're a long way from being able to do things like them.'

The human brain is indeed a wonder. Relative to our size, it's almost twice as large as the brain of any other creature on the planet, and it has immense power. According to one study, to perform the same number of calculations per second as a single human brain, you would need to use every computer in the world.

Part of what makes the human brain unique is the extent of our 'cerebral cortex', the tightly folded layers of neural tissue that give us the skills most other animals lack – the ability to reason, plan and communicate. The cortex is divided into two hemispheres, and each of those into four lobes: the frontal, parietal, temporal and occipital lobes.

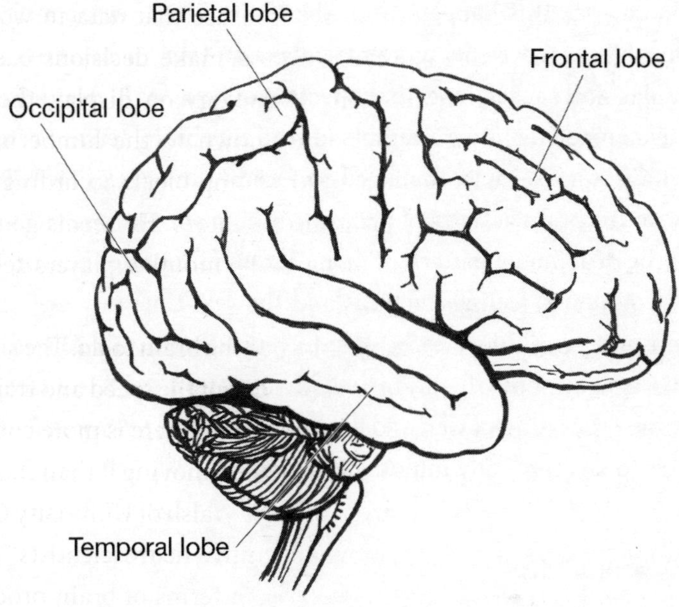

The lobes are made up of neurons. In total, the brain contains up to 100 billion neurons, thin, branching, wire-like cells that carry the electrical and chemical impulses that make you who you are. They both transmit and store information and instructions – they're the internet connection and the hard drive all rolled together.

All a single neuron can do on its own is to fire an electrical impulse along its length, a tiny blip like a flicker of light. But it's the connections that matter: neurons trigger other neurons, and it's the overall pattern of billions of these tiny switches that creates thought and action in response to inputs from the rest of the body.

It's like an orchestra – the overall pattern is not clear until you hear all the instruments playing at once. Or, to use a sporting analogy, imagine the crowd displays you get before kick-off at football matches, where each member of the audience is asked to hold up a piece of coloured card. All one person can do on their own is either hold up their square or not. But bring thousands of people together and they can create pictures or spell out messages.

You can see this happening in the brain. Thinking about a particular object, experiencing a particular emotion, or carrying out a particular skill causes a specific collection of neurons to fire. Scientists have even made tentative attempts to read this brain activity directly. They have, for example, managed to recreate images of faces based solely on the brain activity of people thinking about those faces.

It's the distributed pattern of firing across millions of neurons that creates thoughts, feelings, actions and the real-time processing that Culverhouse would love to be able to reproduce in his robots. This chapter is about how the brains of elite athletes have harnessed that real-time processing power, and how, when applied to vision, it allows athletes to do seemingly impossible things.

Swing and a Miss

An international fast bowler in cricket can deliver the ball at up to 100 miles an hour. At that speed, it takes less than half a second (500 milliseconds) to reach the batsman once it has left the bowler's hand. Given that it takes around 200ms for the batsman's eyes and brain to pick up the flight of the ball, and around 700ms for them to move the bat to intercept the ball, how are batsmen able to hit the thing at all? Professional baseball players and cricketers routinely connect with deliveries that would leave amateurs swinging wildly at empty air, or nursing nasty bruises.

Anticipation is the key to this riddle. Unlike the robots, which only know where the ball is and where it has just been, elite athletes can glean hints as to a ball's likely direction from other sources. Those who seem to have lightning-quick reactions are actually just picking up information that others can't. To prove this, Professor Bruce Abernethy and his colleagues at the University of Queensland have carried out a series of 'occlusion' studies, where they obstruct the vision of batsmen as the ball is being delivered towards them.

It's not quite as dangerous as it sounds.

They use special glasses that turn opaque when triggered by a researcher's laptop or by a foot switch in the bowler's run-up. In one study, six highly skilled and six low skilled batsmen faced three different leg spin bowlers while wearing these glasses, and their vision was shut off (occluded) either just before the ball was released, just before it bounced, or not at all. The more skilled players were much better at hitting the ball without being able to see its full flight, just based on information about the bowler's body and arm movements. Other research has found that international cricket batsmen start moving their feet forwards or backwards before the ball is actually released, while less skilled batsmen tend to wait until its flight path has become more obvious. More recent studies have reduced the visual information even further: skilled batsmen can still predict the path of a ball when shown only the movement of the bowler's joints, or even just a disembodied arm.

It's not just cricket. Abernethy has also asked squash players to predict the direction and force of an opponent's shot from a film display that would cut off right before they played the stroke. Expert squash players were able to pick up more information from the scene than novices. Similar findings have been observed in tennis and football, as technology has made conducting these kinds of experiments more simple. 'It's a hell of a lot easier now,' Abernethy tells me over Skype from his office in Brisbane. When he first started doing experiments like this in the late 1970s, there was no computer editing software to help. 'You'd waste a lot of film trying to get the particular samples you would want,' he says. 'You'd be absolutely petrified that the ball was going to hit the camera, because that would have been a huge expense, and then once you had the footage you had to wait for a week or two for the film to get developed. You then had to go in and deal with physical pieces of film – copy them, splice them together. I spent a good part of my life looking down a low-powered microscope putting little pieces of black plastic on to the film to occlude particular areas.' Things have moved on – from film to digital video to actual cricket and tennis balls coming at people, and beyond to kinematic displays which just show dots of light for the position of the joints. The common theme underlying these experiments remains the same: experts' brains can pick up and act on the smallest pieces of advance information.

Not The Face!

Looking at his goal record for Real Madrid will lead you to one inarguable conclusion: Cristiano Ronaldo can score goals with his eyes shut. On an indoor pitch in a studio in Madrid, the three-time Ballon d'Or winner is putting his skills of anticipation on show for a documentary. First up, though, it's Ronald's turn. Ronald is an amateur footballer; the same age as Ronaldo, but without the requisite skills of anticipation, or the aggressive grooming regime.

He stands inside the area in front of a full-size goal, waiting for former Southend United player and *Soccer AM* presenter Andy Ansah to deliver a cross. As the ball comes in, all the lights in the studio are switched off. A night-vision camera reveals Ronald's bewilderment as he flails and fails to connect with the ball.

Ronaldo does a bit better. He meets the first attempt, in pitch black, with an inch-perfect diving header, and the second with a sweetly struck half-volley into the empty net. 'It's difficult,' he says. 'You have to try and memorise the flight of the ball.' His brain is able to do that extraordinarily quickly; it takes his eyes just 200ms to pick up the information he needs, and his brain only 500ms to calculate the speed and trajectory of the cross and program his body to perform the necessary movements.

For a final test, the experimenters push Ronaldo's anticipatory skills to the limit by switching off the lights even earlier, at the moment the ball is released. All he has to go on is Ansah's body shape as he crosses the ball in. Incredibly, what he does is even better than a diving header or a volley. The ball comes across at head height, but Ronaldo opts to chest it in, propelling it into the bottom corner with a twist of his powerful shoulders. 'This was great,' he says afterwards, grinning. 'I imagine the ball was coming in. I was scared to go with the face, so I go with half chest, half shoulder and put the ball in.'

The best athletes know exactly where to look to get the information they need. Take former FC Barcelona midfielder Xavi, for example, one of the most decorated yet understated footballers of recent years. He was notable not only for his incredibly high pass-completion rate, but also the way he surveyed the pitch, head flicking from left to right like a lizard. 'Some have a mental top speed of 80, while others hit 200,' he has said. 'I try to get close to 200. When a player runs at me, 99 per cent of the time they are stronger than me. So all I can do is think faster.'

This is a trait shared by the world's best passers, as Professor Geir Jordet at the Norwegian School of Sport Sciences discovered when he examined old Premier League footage from Sky Sports' Player Cam – the mode on interactive TV which would follow a single player during the course of a match. He studied the way footballers moved their heads to collect visual information. He watched 118 players across 64 matches, tallying up how many times they turned their gaze away from the ball to pick up information about the position and movement of other players. Two of the league's star midfielders at the time, Frank Lampard and Steven Gerrard, topped the charts in terms of the number of times they looked around the pitch: 0.62 visual searches per second, which is 37 times a minute. Jordet also found a link between the number of visual explorations and pass-completion rates. 'That's what I do: look for spaces,' Xavi told the *Guardian*. 'All day. I'm always looking. All day, all day. Here? No. There? No. People who haven't played don't always realise how hard that is. Space, space, space. I think, the defender's here, play it there. I see the space and pass. That's what I do.'

When we search for objects in our field of view, we don't do it randomly. Research has found that we use contextual cues to help guide our eye movements – we'll look for surfers in the sea, and cars on the road rather than the pavement. Athletes are the same; they adopt unique visual search strategies tailored to their sport.

A study published in the scientific journal *Nature* used head-mounted cameras to measure the eye movements of three cricket batsmen as they faced deliveries from a bowling machine. All three players adopted the same approach. First they looked at the point of delivery: where the ball was about to exit the bowling machine. Then they switched their gaze almost immediately to where the ball was about to bounce. After it bounced, they tracked it for around 200 milliseconds, enough time for their brains to work out where it was going to end up.

The best batsman's eyes were further ahead of the ball. He was able to predict where it would bounce much quicker than the worst player, who took much longer into the ball's initial flight before making an eye movement. This left him unable to play quicker deliveries, because they had already bounced before he had worked out where they were going.

In another experiment for the documentary, Ronaldo and Ansah were fitted with eye-tracking devices – lightweight headgear consisting of a camera and two mirrors. The Real Madrid player tried to keep the ball away from the retired journeyman for five seconds with a series of skills, flicks and moves. The eye-trackers use an infra-red camera to record the movements of the eye, which is then combined with a forward-facing camera feed and some clever software to show exactly where a person was looking at any particular moment. The results are fascinating.

Although Ronaldo glances at the ball frequently as he pulls 13 moves in eight seconds, his eyes are moving around, looking at the defender, scanning the spaces beyond the defender, planning his next move. Ansah's eye movements are all over the place, 'like a pinball', he says, compared to Ronaldo, whose eye movements, or 'saccades', are short, sharp and precise. He looks at the opponent's foot, his other foot or, most importantly, his hips, to pick up advance cues about his future movements.

'[Ronaldo] is effectively a scholar of football,' says sports psychologist Zoe Wilmhurst, who administered the tests. 'It's the same as learning a new language – you build up experience, you learn the basic rules of grammar, in this case the skills, and you put them into the match situation. As you become more fluent you don't need to think about it as much.'

House of Mirrors

The brain of a tennis player returning a first serve has to do three things in about half a second. First, it has to sense that an object is moving towards it dangerously quickly. Second, it has to identify the object and its likely path. Third, it has to decide the best course of action, which in this case is ignoring the natural instinct to dive out of the way, and instead triggering the precise sequence of movements required to direct the object back over the net with the best chance of winning the point.

Over the last few decades, we've discovered more about how athletes' brains learn to do these things by scanning them using fMRI (functional magnetic resonance imaging). Whereas a normal MRI scanner uses powerful magnetic fields to map out the inner health of our joints and organs, or to determine the structure of the brain, an fMRI scanner can measure the flow of blood to different areas of the brain in close to real time.

When people use a particular part of their brain, the neurons in that area use up glucose and oxygen as fuel, and oxygen-rich blood flows into the area to supply more of the raw materials. This oxygenated blood, fresh from the lungs, has different magnetic properties to deoxygenated blood, and an fMRI scanner can detect those differences. Therefore, by putting people in an fMRI scanner while they complete a mental task, we can get a sense of which areas of the brain are being used to complete it.

It's not a direct measure of neural activity because there's a delay of a few seconds between neural activity and blood flow, and also because the clarity of fMRI is not yet good enough to depict things on the minute scale of neurons. But, at the moment, it's the best tool we've got for working out where and how things happen in the brain.

Bruce Abernethy, working with a group from Brunel University London, used fMRI to examine the brains of elite badminton players as they exercised their skills of anticipation. They scanned players of various skill levels as they watched occluded clips of shots being played (the video clips would cut off just before contact was made with the shuttlecock) and tried to predict in which area of the court the shots would land. The expert players showed more brain activity in areas of the brain associated with observing and understanding other people's actions.

One theory is that this activity represents the brain filling in the gaps and creating an 'internal model' – a guess as to what's about to happen based on the movements of the opponent. The more experience an athlete has, the better they are at doing this, and this difference shows up in their brains as well as in their performance.

A few years later, the same group at Brunel did a similar study with footballers, who watched occluded clips of an opponent running towards them with the ball. In some clips, the players would start a feint just before the video cut off, and the footballer in the scanner would have to predict whether they would go left or right. The earlier the clips were cut off, the bigger the difference in neural activity between semi-pro and novice footballers on fMRI scans.

There are cells in the brain called mirror neurons which are specialised for this kind of learning. They were first discovered by chance in the early 1990s by Italian researchers, who observed that the same cells would fire in a monkey's brain when it picked up a piece of food as when it saw a human picking up a piece of food. The presence of mirror neurons has also been detected in humans, who show the same pattern of brain activity when they watch their opponent make a move in a video game as when they make the same move themselves.

About 20 per cent of the neurons in the motor cortex (the area of the brain that controls movement) have this property, and together they've come to be known as the mirror system. 'It's like a virtual reality simulation of the other person's action,' says renowned neuroscientist V.S. Ramachandran, who was one of the first to deliberately study mirror neurons after their accidental discovery. 'The neuron is adopting the other person's point of view.'

A study conducted with basketball players in Rome used a technique called transcranial magnetic stimulation, or TMS, which involves passing a magnetic coil with a current running through it over an area of the brain. It can be used to measure the electrical activity going on inside, or to disrupt it. The researchers showed professional players, coaches and sports journalists occluded clips of the early moments of free throws and asked them to predict whether the throws would be successful or not.

The athletes were better at this, and they were often able to guess correctly even before the ball left the shooter's hands. They also showed a unique pattern of brain activity in the motor cortex. This area of the brain controls movements, but in the case of professional basketball players it was active even when they were just watching free throws on video, and particularly active when they were watching missed shots.

Mirror neurons help the well-trained brains of cricketers, baseball players and footballers to learn from watching their opponents. Combined with their ability to look for visual clues in the right places, this enables them to create more accurate predictions more quickly, and to react at seemingly superhuman speeds.

Eagle Vision

All athletes learn to anticipate through practice and experience, but some of them have innate advantages. Unlike Plymouth's robots, which all have the same brand of camera, not all human eyes are created equal, and that can make a big difference in sport, particularly when it comes to predicting the flight of a ball.

We see when light bounces off objects around us and hits the retina, at the back of the eyeball. The retina consists of a field of cells called rods and cones, which form the sensor of the eye; they react to light, turning it into an electrical signal which is passed down the optic nerve and into the brain. Just as the number of pixels in a digital camera sensor impacts on the sharpness of the pictures it takes, the density of rod and cone cells on the retina can affect the detail with which people are able to see.

In 1996, David Kirschen, Daniel Laby and colleagues tested 387 professional baseball players on their visual acuity – basically, a pixel count for the human optic system. The players were significantly better than the general population: 58 per cent scored 'superior' on the tests, compared to 18 per cent of a control group of non-athletes.

On average, Major League baseball players (excluding pitchers) had a visual acuity of 20/11 in their right eye and 20/12 in their left eye. This means that if the players were looking at an object from 20 feet away, someone with standard 20/20 vision would have to be eight or nine feet closer to it to see it with the same clarity.

Visual acuity is largely determined by the number of rod and cone cells packed on to the retina; this can range from 100,000 to 324,000 per square millimetre. It is thought to be genetic, which means that, in certain sports, players are rising to the top partly because of their innate visual abilities. Another study compared 157 Olympic athletes from different sports, and found that the vision of those from sports such as archery and softball was better than those from track-and-field and boxing. Athletes without the necessary visual equipment may struggle to reach the top level in sports where detailed vision is a big advantage.

Because of their sharper vision, elite baseball players can collect information about the trajectory of objects more easily. In baseball, the movement of the red stitching on the ball gives vital clues about the way a pitch is spinning, which can help batters predict its future flight. Their heightened visual acuity means they can pick up those clues when the ball is further away, giving their brain and body more time to react and play a successful shot. This has been called the 'hardware and software' paradigm. The visual acuity (hardware) of elite athletes makes it easier for them to pick up details, so their brains (the software) have more information to work with in anticipating the ball's flight.

That's not to say that bad eyesight prevents people from reaching sporting greatness, they just might have to develop their skills, or train their software, in a different manner. Cricket batsman Don Bradman – considered one of the greatest ever to play his sport – actually had below average eyesight which prevented him from joining the army during the Second World War. But, unwittingly, he had worked around that as a child by developing his hand-eye co-ordination. He would spend hours practising hitting a golf ball with a cricket stump as it rebounded off a water tank in his family's back yard. 'To me, it was only fun,' he said later. 'But looking back, it was probably a concentrated exercise in accuracy and wonderful training for my eyesight. The golf ball came back pretty fast and I had very little time to get into position for a shot.' Bradman overcame his visual deficit by training his hand-eye co-ordination. He was able to react much later than other players and still play the right shot.

Generally, though, people with naturally good hardware – good visual acuity or depth perception – can train their software much more quickly.

In Plymouth's robots, the distinction between hardware and software is exactly that. They use what Culverhouse calls a 'multi-threaded' approach for their visual processing. The information coming in is analysed in several ways simultaneously to get the quickest results. 'We've got one thread that collects data from the camera and buffers it, and we have other threads consuming data from the camera,' he explains. 'One thread is looking for ball and line markings. Another thread is doing obstacle detection and looking for other robot players.' The human brain does something similar, but it's a bit harder to pinpoint exactly where our hardware ends and our software begins.

The Great Divide

Carbon monoxide is colourless, odourless and toxic to humans. It binds with our red blood cells, preventing them from carrying oxygen to the brain. Without oxygen, neurons die. In the early 1990s, a 35-year-old woman known only as 'DF' suffered carbon monoxide poisoning which left her with two identical brain injuries, or lesions, to the occipital lobes in each hemisphere of her brain. DF is one of the most famous cases in neuroscience because her unique injury revealed that our visual processing is split for efficiency, just as it is in the robots.

Visual processing turns light into information. Your brain builds up a picture of the world around you gradually, starting with neurons in the occipital lobe at the back of the brain that are attuned to very simple features of the world, and then moving up through a hierarchy of increasing complexity.

So, for example, there are neurons in the visual cortex of the brain that fire only when you read particular words. Those neurons will receive inputs from neurons that fire only when you see certain letters. A neuron that responds to seeing the letter H will be triggered to fire by groups of neurons called 'feature detectors' which respond to lines or edges. At the very first level of visual processing there are neurons that respond simply to patches of light or shadow. If you look at a black line on a white background – the middle bar of the letter H, say – a row of those very simple neurons will fire, starting the cascade that turns light hitting the retina into abstract thoughts and concepts.

At all levels, visual processing is organised topographically; adjacent areas of your visual field will activate adjacent areas of the brain. The brain is like a real-time map of your environment and, step by step, it builds up a picture of the world around you, progressing from simple shapes to complex stimuli such as faces and objects.

DF's brain taught us that, at higher levels, visual processing in the brain is split into two streams – one for perception and one for action. The simple feature detector neurons feed into these streams, which consist of a series of closely connected and specialised brain areas.

The ventral stream, or 'what' pathway, helps us recognise objects, shapes and colours, and has strong links with areas of the brain involved in memory. There are neurons high up the ventral stream called grandmother cells, which respond only when you see a specific person.

The dorsal stream handles action. It's also known as the 'where' pathway, and is specialised for processing information about the locations of objects in space and their movements. There are neurons in these areas that respond to linear or circular motion. Other specialised neurons include ones that fire differently depending on the position of your eyes, which could help the brain take into account how your own position is changing relative to an object.

The dorsal stream is also attuned to detect 'optic flow', the way in which the image of an object on your retina changes as it moves. For example, an object getting steadily larger in your visual field is probably coming straight at you, and it might be best to take evasive action. Unless you're a cricketer, in which case you're expected to catch it or hit it, of course.

The carbon monoxide irreversibly damaged the ventral stream – the 'what' pathway – in both hemispheres of DF's brain, which left her unable to recognise objects. She could, however, still perform actions with them, as demonstrated by an experiment in posting letters.

She was able to post a piece of card through an angled slot with no problem whatsoever, but when she was asked to simply align the card with the angle of the slot, she couldn't. Her ventral stream, which guides perception, was damaged, but her dorsal stream, which guides action, was intact.

The dorsal and ventral streams work together in sport. Take tennis as an example. The ventral stream collects information to add context and help guide the decision-making process before the shot is played. The dorsal stream guides the execution of a shot, making sure the ball is hit at the right time and with the right amount of force. It's thought that the ventral stream would be most involved during the early stages of an opponent's shot, gauging things such as body position and racket angle, as well as bringing in information from memory about a particular player's known characteristics. This is all with the goal of helping our player's brain work out whether a cross-court return or an attempt to play a passing shot down the line would be more appropriate. As the opponent actually plays the ball, the dorsal stream jumps in to help guide the action and the successful execution of the return shot.

It is possible that the ventral stream is relied on more by novices, or in unfamiliar situations. One study asked expert golfers to putt with their weaker side. An arrow was placed next to the ball, pointing in the general direction of the hole but slightly rotated away from the correct line for the putt. When putting with their weaker side, golfers tended to be more influenced by the arrow's misleading guidance – their ventral stream was using environmental clues to decide the best course of action. When they tried the same challenge with their usual, stronger side, this effect disappeared. With more automatic and practised movements, the dorsal stream guides action.

Scholes Time

Even at this early stage of cognition, the differences that set elite athletes apart are clear. Whether it's due to practice, innate hardware, or more likely a mixture of both, the brains of athletes in fast ball sports are specialised for anticipation. It's this ability to anticipate and read their sports that seems to give the best athletes all the time in the world.

Perhaps no one epitomises the power and importance of anticipation more than Paul Scholes. The former Manchester United and England midfielder started his career as a short, asthmatic teenager. Like Rooney, Scholes relied on his brain to become one of the greatest players of his generation. Scholes is frequently cited as an inspiration by players like Xavi, Spain's metronomic World Cup winner, for the way he used to drop into space and hit inch-perfect passes over short and long distances. He's used positioning, movement and anticipation to his advantage against players who might be faster, stronger or just bigger, in a compact midfield zone.

This is what his manager Sir Alex Ferguson had to say about him later on in his career: 'He has an awareness of what's happening around him on the edge of the box which is better than most players. As a kid he always had a knack of arriving in the right area just at the right time, but he's proving just as effective from outside the box because he's using his experience in the right way. One of the greatest football brains Manchester United has ever had.'

When I meet him, Scholes has just embarked on a punditry career with BT Sport, where he'll be using his sharpened football mind to analyse matches. It's his last interview of a long day in a meeting room at the BT offices just behind St Paul's Cathedral. The famously reticent man is showing signs of clamming up, but he seems genuinely interested when I tell him about Abernethy's occlusion experiments in other sports. 'That would be difficult,' he muses, as he considers whether he could control a pass without seeing the ball coming towards him. 'There must be some football players who would be able to do that, though – but just to pick the flight of the ball would be incredible.'

The sooner players can pick up the flight of the ball in football, cricket, squash or baseball, the more time they give themselves to decide what to do, and to react. It allows players like Scholes to think several moves ahead. 'The last thing I think about when a ball is coming towards me is where it's going next,' he tells me. He already knows.

Players who can do this well often look like they're playing the game on a different setting to everyone else. I remember going to watch the Portuguese playmaker Luis Figo playing for Inter Milan at the San Siro a few months before he retired. Even though he was the oldest and slowest player on the pitch by far, he always seemed to be in acres of space, never hurried, never rushed. 'When you're playing well, you do feel like you've got all the time in the world,' says Scholes, who had a similar aura on his best days. 'It doesn't feel like that every week,' he adds. 'When you're not playing too well everything can be a bit of a rush and a bit hurried, but when you're playing well you do feel like you've got the pitch to yourself at times.'

This is a phenomenon that has been reported anecdotally across a number of sports, including by F1 drivers when they pull off an overtaking move, and there's compelling evidence that it's more than just a feeling.

Researchers at University College London think the brain has a mechanism for enhancing visual processing when you're preparing to complete an action. They asked volunteers to react to flashing and flickering discs on a screen, either by reaching out to tap the screen, or verbally. The volunteers who had to carry out a physical reaction felt as though they had more time to complete the action than those who weren't asked to move.

'As a midfield player I think the most important thing was always to know where the rest of your team are,' continues Scholes. 'I always tried to have a picture in my head of where my centre forward was, where my wingers were, where the defenders were. You can't just receive a ball and not know what's going to happen or what's around you.'

Scholes echoes Rooney's comments when I ask him to describe his decision-making process as he's receiving a pass and working out what to do with it. 'It depends on where players are on the pitch, where the ball comes in to you. If it's where you want it, can you flick it round the corner to your centre forward? Do you have to take a touch and do it yourself? It's something that's very difficult to explain, but you have the map in your head of where your team are and you take it from there.'

Just like Plymouth's robots, which have a top-down map of the pitch programmed into them, elite footballers are very good at knowing and remembering where their teammates and opponents are on the pitch. Neurons in their hippocampus (a part of the brain important in learning and memory), known as place and grid cells, have become specialised at tracking their position and the locations of their teammates. Everyone has these cells – only a few thousand, but in combination that's enough to code for all the different locations we might find ourselves in during our lives. Place cells are tied to specific locations in the world: when you enter your house, or your office, a specific collection of place cells will be active, and whenever you enter a new place for the first time, a new set of neurons will start firing. Place cells tell you where you are relative to specific landmarks, allowing you to remember where you parked, or navigate around your house in the dark if you're up in the middle of the night. When researchers first discovered place cells in rats in 1971, they were able to tell where an animal was in its cage just by looking at which cells were active. In sport, place cells might be particularly useful for Formula 1 drivers, for example, enabling them to realise when they've reached a particular point in a corner so they know when to brake.

In some sports, like football, athletes can't afford to be constantly scanning around for landmarks to work out their position on the field, which is where grid cells come in. They were first discovered in 2005 by Edvard and May-Britt Moser and John O'Keefe, who shared the Nobel Prize for their work. Grid cells break the world around into triangles, spreading out around you like a carpet made of graph paper.

When you stand on the point of one of these triangles, a particular grid cell will fire, and when you move, say, two steps forward to the point of another triangle, a different grid cell will fire. They mark your place in the world regardless of context, even when you move around. It's how the best athletes always seem to know where the goal is, even when they don't have time to look up; they have an automatic, innate sense of their position because their brains are trained to map space.

Athletes like Scholes combine that information with their skill at picking up clues that can help them anticipate what's going to happen next. In the next chapter, we'll look at how they combine that information with context from other sources to generate ideas about what to do next.

If researchers could have scanned Rooney's brain activity as the ball was coming towards him before that overhead kick, they would have seen a whir of specialised activity just below those expensive hair implants.

That's where information from the place and grid cells is combined with input from memory and vision and feedback from the body, and where the decision about what to do gets made. High-speed decision-making is another area that sets athlete's brains apart, but understanding how and why gives us the opportunity to close the gap.

CHAPTER TWO

MIKA HAKKINEN AND THE ILLUSION OF CHOICE

It is eerily quiet in Greystoke Forest, a stretch of dense pine in England's Lake District criss-crossed by winding gravel tracks. Cutting through the silence like a chainsaw comes the buzz of a petrol engine, and, moments later, the rally car of Elfyn Evans appears, sliding round a bend and throwing up clouds of thick white dust.

The Welshman is the next great hope for British rallying. He has been compared to the legendary Colin McRae, who won two World Rally Championships, and races for the same team: M-Sport.

Greystoke Forest is M-Sport's testing ground, and today Evans is giving journalists a taste of what it is like to be a rally co-driver – one of those hardy folk who sit alongside the driver and give them guidance on what's immediately ahead. Evans has practised on this course plenty of times, so he has no need of the services of an actual co-driver, which is lucky, because with my head being buffeted from side to side with the movement of the car, I doubt I would be able to read anything, let alone the dense and detailed symbols the co-driver translates to tell his partner what is coming up next.

Each pair of driver and co-driver have a preferred system of 'pace notes', honed over years of practice, but a typical example gives the driver the distance to the next corner, the direction and severity of that corner, and details of any hazards such as crests or rocks that need to be watched out for. The instructions for a single corner could be something as simple as '100 K left 2', which is a kink to the left in 100 metres with a severity of '2'. When more detail is added, the instructions can get a bit more complicated. For example, '50 caution jump into right 2 tightens don't cut' signifies that the road rises to a jump 50 metres ahead and then immediately becomes a right-hand bend with a sharpness of '2' which tightens on the exit, and that there's a hazard on the inside so the driver can't cut the corner. There is a lot of information to be transmitted and, during a World Rally Championship stage, the driver and co-driver will work together over a couple of reconnaissance runs to refine and streamline the pace notes.

From the outside, Evans' handling of the car seems perfectly controlled, as he slides around the hairpin we're watching from and accelerates smoothly towards the next bend. Inside the car, it's a completely different story. Strapped in alongside him in the stark, stripped-back interior of his souped-up Ford Focus, it is absolutely frantic. He slams the gearstick and brakes with frightening force, in contrast to the more delicate movements he makes with the steering wheel – constant little adjustments, reacting to changes in grip and slide on an unpredictable surface. The 3-kilometre loop of the forest takes under two minutes, and by the end Evans is red-faced and sweating from both the physical exertion and the concentration.

After the rattle through the woods, I sit down with Evans in M-Sport's impressive headquarters – a 12th-century building that has been converted from a hospital. There's a jarring contrast between the original stonework of Dovenby Hall and the vast, spotless warehouse extension where the construction work on the team's rally cars takes place.

Evans looks much younger than his 27 years, but despite his boyish features he carries himself in the determined manner of an experienced racer, even though it's only his first full year in the World Rally Championship. Prominent ears stick out either side of a shock of short brown hair, and his bright blue eyes slowly scan the opulent surroundings as he considers my questions. In an ornate dining room that clashes spectacularly with the bright blue of Evans' branded racing overalls, I ask him what is going through his head when he's driving at race pace. His answer is surprising.

'The honest truth is nothing,' he says in his soft Welsh patter. 'Very few times do you actually have many thoughts in the car when you're driving, because things happen so quickly. You just have to let it come naturally. Yes, there are areas of thought at some point, but you tend to find that when you perform at your best you come to the stage where you don't really know what you've thought about for the last 15 to 20 minutes.'

However, even though Evans might not be aware of it, his brain is still making hundreds of decisions a second. Consider all the things it has to calculate and take into account when he steers round a corner. First, it has to process the information coming in from his eyes about his current speed and position on the road. Then, from his limbs and the rest of his body, he'll get a sense of how the car is gripping the road as it approaches the corner, and whether he needs to make any adjustments to account for that. Then, unique to rallying, he'll also be processing the information relayed to him by the co-driver, which Evans will combine with his own memories from previous events at the same course, his assessment of the prevailing conditions, and his knowledge of the best or fastest line to take through the corner. During a competitive event, his brain will also be factoring in information relayed to him by his team about how his rivals are doing, whether he should take a gamble and push to gain time, or play it safe and consolidate his position.

This all happens before he has even started steering or braking to take the corner. Even a simple decision about how much to turn the wheel or press the throttle requires the brain to weigh up dozens of different sources of information in a split second, carry out complex calculations, and spit out an answer that is quick enough, accurate enough and flexible enough to cope with changing conditions. As the number of variables increases, the complexity rises exponentially, and this is something that is true across all sports. This chapter is about how athletes make sense of the whirlwind of information that surrounds them, and how they use it to make quick and accurate decisions.

Even doing something that seems relatively simple like controlling a football or catching a cricket ball requires calculating the trajectory of an object moving at speed, changing one's own direction to meet it, and then making movements precise enough to connect with it in such a way that it doesn't simply bounce away. This requires an immense amount of processing power, which is one of the many reasons why Mustachio and his robotic teammates won't be beating Real Madrid any time soon.

The robot footballers at the University of Plymouth have a memory chip which stores all the information they need for working out what to do next. The chip, says Phil Culverhouse, 'maintains a real-time copy of everything that is happening, including all the sensor input from the robot, where they think the ball is, where they think the goal is, and all the sensor input from all the other robots so any individual robot can make a decision about what it is going to do next'.

The human system is quite similar. But even the remarkable brains of athletes don't have infinite processing power. There's only so much information we can hold in our heads at any one time; only so much capacity in our own memory chips. Psychologists call this concept 'working memory', and have used many different analogies to explain it over the years. In the 1950s, it was thought of as a blackboard, but now the best analogy is probably the RAM on a computer. Our working memory holds all the information we need to perform whatever task it is we're currently trying to complete.

In the 1950s, a Princeton psychologist called George Miller

published his discovery that the average person can only hold between five and nine items in their working memory. This average of 7+/-2 became known as Miller's Law, and it holds true across a number of different categories. You can try it with numbers. Look at this list and then cover it up for about 10 seconds and see how many you can recall in order.

58201230719662742015

People use different strategies to try to remember a list like that. A lot will try to repeat the numbers back to themselves in their head, as you might do when you're trying to retain a phone number while looking for a pen. As per Miller's Law, most people will be able to remember around seven items and then struggle. That's just one fairly straightforward set of information. Determining the correct course of action in a sport such as rallying requires taking into account hundreds of interlocking variables, and making the calculations to execute those actions accurately. It's certainly more than seven bits of information.

So, are the brains of elite athletes like Elfyn Evans different? Do they have a bigger working memory capacity to allow them to make all the calculations they need to, or more processing power to churn through them more quickly? The answer is usually no. But the brains of elite sportspeople have developed unique processing strategies to help them perform.

On Fire With The Flying Finn

The brake discs are on fire. Mika Hakkinen has just come screeching into the pits at Silverstone in a Mercedes AMG, and he has been driving the car so hard that the carbon fibre pads that apply friction to the tyres have actually ignited. The two-time Formula 1 world champion steps out of the car in black leathers, which are bulging slightly more than they did at the peak of his career, ruffles his blond hair and casts an amused look at a technician rushing forward with a fire extinguisher. There is much mirth from many of the watching crowd, here for a media day with one of McLaren's sponsors, but not from me. It's my turn next.

After a short break to let the car cool down a bit, I join the Finnish driver for a blast around Silverstone's famous circuit. He is driving on the absolute edge – tyres screeching, throwing up smoke, engine roaring in our ears. At one point he actually pushes it a bit too far and starts to slide into the gravel. You might expect absolute concentration from someone pushing a highly tuned machine to its limits at speed, as we saw from Elfyn Evans earlier. But, instead, Hakkinen is laughing and joking. 'This is how I drive my family to the shops!' he shouts over the engine's throaty growl, before glancing at the in-car radio and asking whether I want him to put on some music. I do not.

The reason Hakkinen is able to hold a conversation while zooming around a circuit at speed is because he has had years of practice, and that practice has changed the way his brain works. Instead of being handled by the conscious parts of his brain, all the complex decisions and movements required to handle the car and select the right braking points and steering angles have been outsourced to the subconscious regions.

The decisions have become automatic, freeing up areas of the brain involved in more conscious thought to focus on higher concerns – in this case, terrifying journalists.

The road to this kind of automaticity starts with chunking. Chunking is reminiscent of the process of refinement a rally driver and his co-driver go through with the pace notes before a stage. It is taking information and grouping it in a way that makes it easier to process. Think back to the numbers I asked you to remember just before. Now try the same numbers again, but 'chunked' into a format we're more familiar with.

5/8/2012, 30/7/1966, 27/4/2015

They are dates of course. In this case the dates of Super Saturday for Great Britain at the London Olympics, England winning the World Cup, and AFC Bournemouth effectively sealing their promotion to the Premier League. You were likely able to apply your knowledge of date formats to the data to break it into more meaningful sections. The 7+/-2 limit of Miller's Law still applies, but you have circumvented it by turning 20 bits of information into just three.

In the 1960s, a Dutch chess player and psychologist called Adriaan de Groot ran an innovative experiment where he showed chess masters and less skilled players chess pieces arranged on a board. After five seconds, he took the pieces away and asked the participants to reconstruct the layout from memory. The masters were much better at doing this, but only when the pieces had been configured in an arrangement that you might see in a real game of chess. Instead of simply seeing the pieces arranged randomly as a non-expert might, they broke them down into a meaningful chunk, the same way you might break up a string of letters into words, or a string of numbers into dates.

Chunking lets experts process the same amount of information while using fewer mental resources, and they do it automatically. Another study of chess players showed them a layout and asked them to recreate it on another board. The experts needed fewer glances at the first board to put the pieces in the right place than novices did.

The same thing has also been observed in more athletic pursuits.

As Liverpool's great team of the late 1980s and early 1990s were unravelling, to be knocked off their perch by a Manchester United side that included Scholes, researchers from the two rival cities were collaborating to test the spatial abilities of football players. They showed players 10-second video sequences of games. The clips were either structured – for example, the build-up of an attack through passing; or unstructured – the somewhat chaotic arrangement of players following a rebound or a turnover in possession. Experienced players were much better at remembering the positions of specific players in structured clips than inexperienced players were, but this advantage disappeared for unstructured clips.

American football players needed fewer looks at a formation layout to recall it accurately; they too chunked it into larger pieces, resulting in fewer bits of information to remember. High school American football coaches were able to fill in a playing scene accurately without even having seen the whole thing. They were shown limited information, but were able to use their sporting knowledge to work out what category of play they were looking at and fill in the gaps. Where a non-expert might see a seemingly random assortment of players, experts see and think in patterns.

The way that coaches and quarterbacks in American football communicate which plays they want their players to run is another vivid example of chunking in sport. It can cause problems when players change teams, as former NFL quarterback Trent Dilfer told now defunct sports website FanHouse in a piece about the different strategies players adopt to memorise the complex and intricate sequences. 'A lot of coaches use numbering systems,' he said. 'Red Right 22 Texas is a West Coast play. In another system it's Split Right Scat Right 639 F Angle.'

The way that we describe formations in football is a simpler form of chunking: 4-4-2 or 4-3-3 describes the position of 10 outfield players on the pitch, turning 10 bits of information into just three. Like the pace notes used by the rally drivers, elite sportspeople have structures in place to break down complicated information into chunks that are easier to remember, freeing up their mental resources and attention. For Dilfer, there's a difference between just learning a play and 'owning it'. 'Owning it to me goes from knowing it, to understanding it, to it becoming instinctive,' he said.

Automatic, Systematic, Hydromatic

Chunking isn't confined to abstract things such as numbers or positions. It also happens whenever you learn a new skill. The first time Evans got into a car his movements would have been slow and deliberate, just like anyone learning to drive. He would have found it difficult to focus on steering and changing gear at the same time, or lifting the clutch and pressing the throttle simultaneously to find the biting point.

It's the same for everyone. When we're first learning to do something, we may know what we're meant to do but it's hard to hold everything we need in our heads; we find it difficult to remember how to change from second to third gear while also remembering to put our foot on the clutch, check our mirrors and keep the car on the road. With practice, the skills undergo a process of chunking, becoming more and more automatic. We start 'owning them'.

Two American researchers, Matthew Smith and Craig Chamberlin, demonstrated this when they asked a group of footballers to dribble through a slalom course, and then repeat it while simultaneously keeping an eye on a screen on the wall to look out for when a particular shape appeared on it. The novice players really suffered. Their times were much slower because their brains couldn't handle the load of completing both tasks together. But the experts were almost as quick as they had been before, even with this extra task added.

You can see this change from conscious to automatic control happening in an fMRI scanner. Researchers at Stanford University in California scanned people's brains while they completed a reaction-time task, and found that the brain was initially active in a wide range of areas, but as people learnt how to do the task, the activity in those areas decreased. This is something we'll revisit later in the book – elite athletes' brains tend to run more 'quietly' than those of non-experts.

Further down the California coast at the University of Santa Barbara, Nicholas Wymbs tapped into the neural processes underlying motor chunking, the process by which physical skills become automatic. 'You can think about a chunk as a rhythm,' he said, referring to the pattern of sequences and pauses when we're learning something new, whether it's a gap between the first and second part of a phone number or between the component parts of a tennis serve.

To start with, the prefrontal cortex is heavily involved. This hugely important area is right at the front of the brain and it is involved in a wide range of higher mental functions, from attention and working memory to personality and social behaviour. It also helps us break down a complex skill into more manageable pieces when we're learning it. You might break down a tennis serve into the ball toss, the swing and getting set for the return, for example. But in order to make everything automatic, the brain needs to knit those individual pieces back together into a fluid whole. Wymbs and his colleagues scanned people's brains while they tapped out a sequence of keys based on some notation in front of them, almost like playing a piano or the guitar (or the video game *Guitar Hero*). 'After practising a sequence for 200 trials, they would get pretty good at it,' he said. 'After a while, the note patterns become familiar. At the start of the training, it would take someone about four and a half seconds to complete each sequence of 12 button presses. By the end of the experiment, the average participant could produce the same sequence in under three seconds.'

The brain scans revealed that a deep and primitive part of the brain called the basal ganglia took over as tapping out the sequence became more automatic. It's almost as if automaticity is cutting out the middle man; like a new employee being trained, once the basal ganglia has been told what to do and repeated it enough times, it can complete the task on its own without supervision from the higher areas of the brain. In fact, like said employee when their boss is breathing down their neck, performance can often suffer when the conscious brain tries to take over again. Athletes can end up overthinking something they usually do without conscious thought, and as a result their movements revert to those of a novice – jerky, unco-ordinated and disastrous. This is one of the classic mechanisms of choking under pressure and it's something we'll delve into in more depth in a later chapter. One study illustrates the importance of automaticity particularly well, however.

Two economists at the University of Pennsylvania, Devin Pope and Maurice Schweitzer, analysed over 2.5 million golf putts from various levels of competition, and discovered that professional golfers were less accurate when putting for birdie than they were when trying to make par, regardless of the distance or difficulty of the putt. When players were on the verge of improving their score, their attention was drawn to their movements and the conscious part of the brain started interfering. Something that should have been an easy, automatic task reverted to the insurmountable feat of co-ordination it seems like on the surface.

When a novice cricketer starts to run in to bowl, he'll be thinking about the grip of the ball in his hand, hitting the crease without putting his foot over it, timing the leap to maximise the momentum of his bowling arm, and keeping that arm as straight as possible. His prefrontal cortex will be buzzing with variables and information.

When a more experienced player runs in, he will not be thinking about any of that. His basal ganglia will have taken over control of the bowling action. If he is thinking at all, it will be about where he is going to pitch the ball, the weaknesses of the batsman at the other end, and how this delivery fits into the sequence he's going to use to try to get the batsman out.

It is not possible for the limited capacity of our working memory to consciously handle all the variables required to bowl accurately at speed, or hit a tennis return, or pull off an overhead kick. But when the processes become so automatic that we don't even have to think about them, we can do things that at first seemed impossible, and we can do them in the face of all kinds of distractions.

'You Get The Decision Made'

'When a cross comes into a box, there are so many things that go through your mind in a split second, like five or six different things you can do with the ball,' is how Wayne Rooney describes his decision-making process in that *ESPN* magazine interview from the introduction. 'You get the decision made,' he continued. 'Then it's obviously about the execution.'

To get the decision made, the brain needs to take into account information from a number of different sources, generate potential options, and weigh up the risks and rewards of each one before making a choice. To find out how it does it, I got in touch with an old friend for a bit of help. Dr Nils Kolling was my tutorial partner at university and he still works in the imposing concrete block that is Oxford University's Experimental Psychology department, where he conducts research into how the brain makes decisions and weighs up risk.

'This is a very interesting question, especially in regards to people with high degrees of expertise such as professional athletes,' he says. 'The shortest answer is that the brain makes decisions using a variety of different systems depending on the particular situation at hand. Every decision-making system and its corresponding neural structures have their own specification, advantages and disadvantages, competing with each other constantly to drive behaviour.'

There are at least three systems, 'but probably more', and it's likely that athletes switch between them pretty fluidly while performing their sports.

The first group are the slower, harder decisions, the kind we all have to make regularly at work and in our personal lives. Think of a football manager surveying the transfer market and choosing between a flashy winger or a solid centre half, or a tennis coach trying to work out what advice to give a player being battered by his opponent's powerful backhand. An area at the bottom of the frontal lobe called the ventromedial prefrontal cortex (vmPFC) is involved in evaluating various options according to a number of different criteria. 'For example, when buying a house you might consider its price, location and a million other factors to come to a single simple desirability index or universal currency value and pick accordingly,' says Kolling. 'The vmPFC is the area that allows you to do so, and without it people sometimes make inconsistent decisions.'

The second group are automatic decisions, things such as how to control a pass in football, which as we've seen are often associated with subcortical, more evolutionarily basic structures including the basal ganglia. 'A lot of these things might not even look like decisions anymore,' says Kolling.

For sport, though, the most interesting kinds of decisions are in a third group that fall somewhere in between the automatic processes and the slower deliberations, and they change depending on the context of the game. 'A decision might not exclusively be based on the specific values of particular courses of action or options, but instead requires you to use a vague or general sense of the environment you find yourself in,' explains Kolling. 'For example when deciding whether to engage with a specific task you might compare it to a specific alternative, or instead, with your sense of whether there are better things to do elsewhere, even though you have nothing else specific in mind. This allows you to forage or search for better things, when you know you are in a generally rich environment, rather than getting stuck with comparatively bad options.'

So, for example, a Formula 1 driver might decide not to attack at a particular corner to try to overtake, in the expectation that a better opportunity will come along later in the race. Kolling and his colleagues at Oxford have found evidence that an area of the frontal cortex is involved in making these kinds of decisions, and bringing in context from the environment. 'For example, it could allow you to take risks flexibly if the situation is such that there is large pressure towards or against taking risks,' he says. 'A football player during the last minutes of a losing game is a great example of this. During that time he will weigh up risks and rewards very differently than he would during the start of the game.'

At a neural level, the mechanism for making a decision is a democracy. Take Rooney's overhead kick, for instance. The player's brain generates action plans such as 'bring the ball down on the chest' or 'head it first time' in a wide range of brain regions across the frontal and parietal lobes. The options are represented by the distributed pattern of electrical activity in the neurons – remember the crowd holding up different-coloured cards to make an image.

Electrical impulses from different areas of the brain act like voters, feeding into the different potential choices. These inputs come from areas like the dorsal stream, which processes information about the position of objects, from place and grid cells, which provide information about location and space, and from the nerves of the muscles and joints. They can either be excitatory or inhibitory – like 'yes' or 'no' votes in a referendum, neurons can make the neurons they're connected to either more or less likely to fire. This is how the brain takes into account information from various sources when making all kinds of choices.

All these inputs from across the brain and body add to and subtract from the different action plans, and when the level of electrical activity (called the decision variable) in the neurons representing one of the options reaches a certain threshold, the brain initiates that action. The decision is made.

But the brain's work does not end there. Even after an action has been decided on and initiated, the brain needs to constantly adjust its instructions based on feedback from the body and other senses. The brain starts by setting a goal – 'head the ball', for example – and makes predictions about what kind of feedback it should get from the eyes and body if it is on track to achieve that goal.

If the actual sensation and information from the world doesn't match the prediction, the brain can revise its action plan to reduce the error. 'The brain does not merely issue rigid commands,' writes science journalist Carl Zimmer in *Discover* magazine, 'it also continually updates its solution to the problem of how to move the body. Athletes may perform better than the rest of us because their brains can find better solutions than ours do.'

Cutting Mental Corners

When a baseball leaves a bat, there are myriad factors determining where it will go, including the force of the batter's swing, the angle of contact, the spin on the pitch, humidity in the air and wind direction.

An elite fielder looking to catch that ball has already given themselves an edge. They will have used their experience to watch the right areas, so they will know what kind of thing to expect before a non-professional would know. Their motor movements will be automatic, so the process of actually catching the ball shouldn't be too taxing, providing they don't overthink it.

However, their brain still has to work out where the ball is going to land, which in theory means calculating its trajectory and speed. Slight changes in speed can make a big difference, but the only information fielders have is what their eyes can give them.

They can't measure wind speed, and they don't have physics training. If you gave them a maths problem on paper asking them to calculate the trajectory of a ball, most would struggle. But, despite that, they take just a fraction of a second to start running for the ball.

The brain is adept at using shortcuts to solve problems like this. Also called 'schemas' or 'heuristics', these shortcuts are unconscious processing strategies which, like chunking, help reduce the load on our cognitive machinery. In *Thinking Fast and Slow,* Nobel Prize winner Daniel Kahneman describes a heuristic as 'a simple procedure that helps find adequate, though often imperfect, answers to difficult questions'. It's a rough calculation, a rule of thumb.

Peter McLeod of Oxford University and Zoltan Dienes of Sussex University used a bowling machine to test what approach skilled fielders in cricket use when they're catching the ball. They set the machine to fire balls up in the air at different speeds so they would land at different distances from a fielder, either in front of them or behind them. They measured the running speed and direction of the fielders as they tried to intercept the ball and found that they ran in such a way as to keep the angle of their gaze on the ball constant throughout its flight.

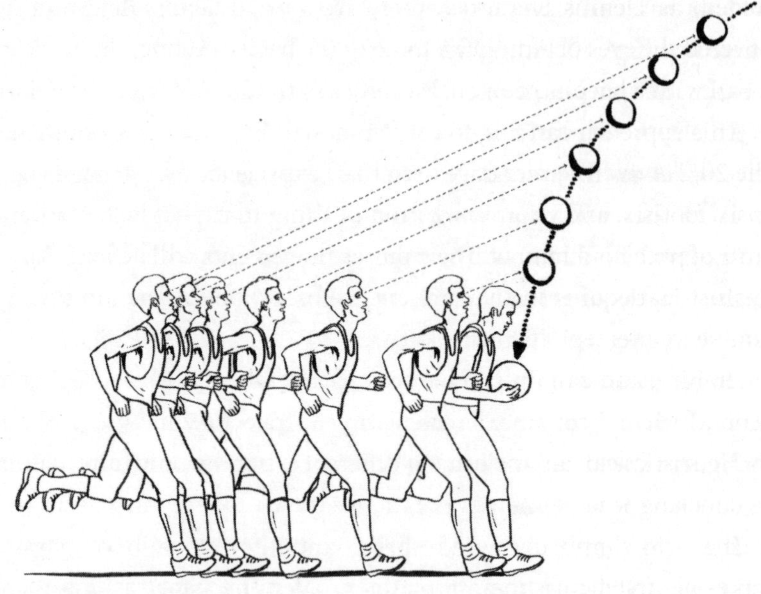

Fielders' brains don't calculate trajectory or wind speed or anything that would tax their working memory. By simply keeping their eyes on the ball and adjusting the speed of their movements so that their gaze stays at the same angle to the ball, they will inevitably intercept it just as it reaches catching height. We've already seen how there are neurons in the visual cortex of our brains specialised for things like optic flow, the way the size of an object changes on our retina as it moves away or towards us. It's quite possible that experienced catchers have highly trained neurons that take into account the angle of their eyes when they focus on a moving object.

Mental shortcuts like this have been called 'fast and frugal heuristics', because they're quick and they don't require complicated or precise calculations. Another example is the constant-angle strategy, which covers intercepting an opponent's run, for example in rugby or American football. Athletes employ the same approach as a lion attacking a speeding gazelle – they run towards where the target will be. This is so ingrained in athletes that they even do it while blindfolded, as Dennis Shaffer at Ohio University discovered when he covered the eyes of American footballers and asked them to intercept a ball with a beeping device inserted into it.

This approach can fall down at times, as Harlequins found out in the 2013 Aviva Premiership final. Leicester Tigers flanker Tom Croft is six-foot-six, and weighs more than 17 stone, but he has a surprising turn of pace for a man of his build and his position. Watching his try against Harlequins in that game, you can see the defender setting a course to intercept, but because of Croft's surprising speed he doesn't catch him, and can only graze his ankles as he runs over the line to score.

Heuristics can also be used as shortcuts to sporting decisions, such as choosing who to pass to. The least mentally taxing way of selecting a pass is to simply choose the first option you think of. This is the 'take-the-first' heuristic, and there's evidence across basketball, Aussie Rules and handball that this is what athletes do between 60 and 90 per cent of the time.

This is due to the order in which options are generated, and how it changes based on previous experience. 'Options that are repeatedly used in previous similar situations develop stronger links,' says Markus Raab, who has led the work on sporting heuristics. 'The take-the-first heuristic simply "bets" that these earlier-generated options are better.' Research also indicates that expert athletes actually generate fewer options than non-experts; they're able to select the best option so quickly that they don't need to generate many alternatives.

One of the leading theories about how experts are able to make high-speed decisions so quickly and accurately is another mental shortcut – making decisions on the basis of familiar patterns or cues from the environment. This has been written about a lot. It's been called System 1 thinking by Daniel Kahneman in *Thinking Fast and Slow*, in contrast to slower, more effortful System 2 thinking. It's an idea that has also been explored by Malcolm Gladwell in *Blink*, but both writers owe much to the work of Gary Klein, who named it the 'recognition-primed decision model'.

'Experts see things that the rest of us cannot, often experts do not realise that the rest of us are unable to detect what seems obvious to them,' he wrote in his book *Sources of Power*. He uses the examples of firefighters intuitively knowing when a burning building is about to collapse, but the same principle is true of athletes as well.

'Experts should be more sensitive to the right pieces of information,' says Kolling, which is something we've already seen from their powers of anticipation and knowing where to look. Cristiano Ronaldo knows where the defender is about to go because he knows to look at the movement of his hips to collect the relevant information.

The simplest model of recognition-primed decision-making involves the athlete performing a particular action or making a particular decision in response to a specific stimulus. In baseball, recognition-primed decision-making might mean swinging in a particular way (or not swinging at all) when you see the pattern of spin or the movement of a pitcher's arm associated with a curveball or a slider. In football, it might mean making a run to the near post when you see a winger's head go down before he whips in a cross.

Athletes match what they're experiencing to situations they've previously encountered in a game or in training, and then make the appropriate choice based on their experience. The purpose of training is to increase the athletes' well of experience of different stimuli, so they'll know the right decision to make in any situation, to make the unpredictable world of sport predictable.

These intuitive decisions are generally correct. One study of elite chess players found that forcing them to rush through their moves barely impaired their performance at all, because they were normally right first time.

Over time these decision circuits are trained through experience, and complex choices become instinct or intuition. Athletes feel like they're guessing, but most of the time they're right. Every time they make a pass or hit a six, they get faster and more accurate as their brain physically changes. This is neural plasticity and, as we'll discover in the next chapter, it is the key to understanding what makes the athletic brain unique.

CHAPTER THREE

ROGER FEDERER AND THE CHANGING BRAIN

Billy Morgan's heart is racing. It is April 2015 and on the slopes of Livigno in the Italian Alps the 26-year-old snowboarder is about to attempt a world first. There is very little margin for error.

'We'd been thinking about it for six months,' Morgan tells me when I interview him later that year. 'I'd been worrying about it and losing sleep over it for ages, never thinking that the day would actually come that I would have to go and do it.'

Southampton-born Morgan has mid-length, dirty-blond hair parted in the middle and tucked behind his ears, and deep blue eyes. He looks like a forgotten member of Nirvana. He is one of the best snowboarders in the world, and finished 10th in the slopestyle event at the 2014 Winter Olympics in Sochi, a discipline where competitors are judged on their ability to pull off jaw-dropping aerial tricks.

The backside 1800 quad cork is suitably spectacular – a breathtaking stunt involving four mid-air rotations. 'It was a big step,' explains Morgan. 'No one had done four rotations yet, so it upped the level again. It was pretty big, and there's not a lot of other sports where they go upside down four times.'

Successfully landing a trick like the quad cork requires an extraordinary combination of power, co-ordination, bravery and awareness. The power comes from Morgan's muscles, built up through years of training. Co-ordination and the rest come from his brain, which, like a muscle, has also been changed through the years of practice.

'What needs to be trained well is the autopilot,' says Morgan. 'If your autopilot doesn't work then it can go bad. It's about knowing when to come out – when to open up to put your landing down. A split second too early and you're upside down. But that just comes from doing it heaps. You watch people try and double cork the first time, and you can tell somebody that's got good aerial skill from somebody that's just going for it, because they're just like a bag of lettuce being thrown in the air. There's no change in body shape because they haven't experienced it before, and really they shouldn't be doing it. They should be practising their general aerial awareness so they've got body control in the air.'

Morgan has built his repertoire from smaller chunks, learning to nail the take-off, and then the landing, and then piecing it all together. Like rally driver Elfyn Evans, Morgan says that there's nothing really going through his head when he's executing a complicated move. 'I've come to the conclusion that there's too much information for your body to be able to remember,' he says. 'You're concentrating so much that when you've landed you've forgotten what was going on before.'

Anders Ericsson has devoted his life to learning how people like Morgan have developed their expertise. He grew up in Sweden, and started his scientific career at a time of great sporting success for the Scandinavian country: Ingemar Stenmark was dominating the world of skiing, and tennis star Bjorn Borg was winning title after title at Wimbledon and the French Open. Ericsson, whose interest stemmed from his own failures at the chessboard, would go on to shape the way we understand expertise in sport, music and beyond.

His research spawned the now famous '10,000-hour rule' – the idea that you can become an expert at anything with 10,000 hours of deliberate practice. Whether it's a language, an instrument, a sport, or something more abstract like software development, proponents of the theory argue that practice is the only thing that separates the best from the rest. Although Ericsson himself believes his work has been misinterpreted, the rule stems from a study in which he asked violinists of varying skill levels what age they had started playing at, how many hours a day they practised, and how many hours a day they thought they had put in to playing the violin up to that point in their life. The best group – those who were rated as having the potential to become world-class soloists – had reached an average of 10,000 hours of practice.

It's an idea that captures the imagination, particularly for anyone who has ever struggled through PE lessons at school, or fumbled their way through 'Wonderwall' on an acoustic guitar. The idea that you can be as good as your heroes if you just put enough work in is powerful and persuasive. It's what convinced would-be golfer Dan McLaughlin to quit his job as a photographer at the age of 31 and pursue 10,000 hours of practice with the goal of joining the PGA Tour. He is due to reach his target in October 2016.

It is also indicative of a seismic paradigm shift that has taken place in neuroscience, particularly in the last 40 years or so: a move away from the notion that people are born with innate mental talents. In the early 19th century, the early days of the science, phrenology was one of the most popular modes of thinking about the brain.

This theory depicted the brain as being made up of specific modules dedicated to different thoughts or emotions. It was believed that you could measure aspects of a person's character by taking precise measurements of their skull in different areas. You might have seen the ceramic skulls, now sold as household ornaments, marked in a grid with different areas labelled with vague terms such as 'intuition' or 'foresight'.

Nowadays, neuroscientists see the brain as fluid, flexible and malleable, as much a product of nurture as nature. Of course, there is still a genetic component to sporting success; you are unlikely to make it to the 100 metres final at the Olympics if you don't have the right kind of fast-twitch muscle fibres, no matter how many hours of practice you put in. We saw in chapter one how success as a baseball batter was closely correlated with the innate visual acuity of the retina, which had an impact on the athlete's ability to read the spin on the ball at an early stage of the pitch.

Even if commentators and fans still talk about natural talent and gifted individuals, scientists now tend to look at experts as a product of practice rather than providence. Or at least, as Malcolm Gladwell argues in *Outliers,* expertise is viewed as a product of the *opportunity* to have practised for more than 10,000 hours, which still often owes something to environment and chance.

Look at Rory McIlroy, who was chipping golf balls into washing machines on Irish television at the age of six, or tennis champions Serena and Venus Williams, whose father Richard created a 78-page dossier when they were children outlining his plan to get them to the top of the women's game.

Athletes aren't born with the ability to read the bounce of a cricket ball, or make quick and accurate decisions in a split second. They learn through thousands of hours of practice. All that practice changes the brain, because everything you do changes your brain. When Morgan snowboards down a hill or over a jump, he's leaving as much of an impression on his own mind as he leaves in the snow that he carves through.

This is neural plasticity. It means our minds are malleable, like Plasticine. It allows our brains to be flexible, to learn from new experiences and to adapt and recover from injuries. Everything we do and experience shapes our brain in some minuscule way. Over time, the changes add up, altering how we'll behave in the future, just as the tracks Morgan leaves in the snow will create a slightly different experience for the next person to tackle the same slope.

'The plastic brain is like a snowy hill in winter,' explains plasticity pioneer Alvaro Pascual-Leone, quoted in Norman Doidge's excellent book *The Brain That Changes Itself.* 'Aspects of that hill – the slope, the rocks, the consistency of the snow – are, like our genes, a given. When we slide down on a sled, we can steer it and will end up at the bottom of the hill by following a path determined both by how we steer and the characteristics of the hill. Where exactly we will end up is hard to predict because there are so many factors in play. "But," Pascual-Leone says, "what will definitely happen the *second time* you take the slope down is that you will more likely than not find yourself somewhere or another that is related to the path you took the first time. It won't be exactly that path, but it will be closer to that one than any other. And if you spend your entire afternoon sledding down, walking up, sledding down, at the end you will have some paths that have been used a lot, some that have been used very little . . ."'

If you're reading this as an adult who still daydreams about making it as an athlete, and you don't want to quit your job like Dan McLaughlin, the good news is that our growing knowledge of neural plasticity could help break the 10,000-hour rule. Understanding how practice has changed the brains of elite athletes can help amateurs improve their game, and is helping scientists and start-ups develop new brain-training tools to push the boundaries of human performance. But to understand them, first you need to understand how years of graft can change the way you think. In explaining, I'll touch on Roger Federer's giant hands, Andy Cole and Dwight Yorke's beautiful friendship, and the terrifying prospect of neural doping. But this journey starts, as plenty do, in the back of a London taxi.

Use It Or Lose It

It's painted purple. And I've just seen what I think was a severed cow's head by the side of the road. But other than that, I could be driving down Clapham High Street. I am in the back of a classic London cab, although it's one of several hundred that have been sprayed a rich hue and shipped over to Baku, the capital of Azerbaijan, ahead of the 2015 European Games. The taxi driver, who currently has more passengers than remaining teeth, certainly has plenty of life experience, but I'm not sure whether he has amassed his 10,000 hours of driving experience given the alarming way we're bouncing along a dirt road on the outskirts of the oil-rich city.

A neuroscientist armed with an fMRI scanner would be able to tell that something wasn't quite right with our London cab, because black cabbies in the English capital were one of the first groups to demonstrate how practice can change your brain. To get their licence, even in this age of sat-navs and Uber, each has to pass a stringent test called The Knowledge, which involves memorising vast swathes of London's intricate road layout.

All this learning has been found to change the size of the hippocampus, an area of the brain that encodes spatial relationships and memory. It's much larger in London taxi drivers than in normal people, and its size has been found to be correlated with the number of years cabbies have spent in the job.

As brain-imaging techniques have developed over recent decades, neuroscientists have learnt more about what's happening inside your head when you practise. In some ways, the brain behaves just like a muscle. When you use it, it grows, and when you don't, it shrinks. Maybe the phrenologists weren't completely wrong after all.

Bulging biceps aren't the only things that can identify an elite athlete. Golfers come in all shapes and sizes, but their neural architecture might give them away to a perceptive neuroscientist. In 2009, a team of researchers in Switzerland replicated Ericsson's initial research into violinists, but with a group of 40 men who had varying levels of golf skill and experience. Ten of the group were professionals, 10 had a handicap of between zero and 14, 10 had a handicap of between 15 and 36, and the final 10 had never played a game of golf in their life, not even mini-golf (in golf the lower the handicap, the better the player).

Instead of taking the last group down to the pitch-and-putt for a long overdue session, the researchers instead asked the other three groups when they'd started playing golf, and how many hours in total they thought they had played up until that point in their life. It won't surprise you that the professionals had started at a much younger age than the other two groups. But the biggest difference was in the total number of hours they had spent playing. The worst group averaged 758 hours of total golf time, the middle group had managed to rack up 3,207 hours of golf on average, while the professionals had amassed a staggering average of 27,415 hours of golf.

To put that into perspective: if you played for eight hours a day, every day, including weekends and public holidays, it would take you almost 10 years to clock up that many hours. The professional group had managed to amass this much practice by an average age of 31.

All this practice had changed them dramatically, as the Swiss researchers found when they scanned the golfers' brains to look for changes in grey matter, which is made up of neurons and their branches. The golfers in the best two groups had more grey matter volume than the others in a network of brain areas across the frontal and the parietal lobes – areas involved in the control of movements.

These areas of the brain had literally grown bigger with practice.

Chinese scientists found similar results when they compared the brains of professional divers with those of non-divers. Areas of the cortex were thicker in several areas in the divers, including a part of the brain known to play an important role in the perception of biological motion. The researchers, from the Chinese Academy of Science in Beijing, believe that the increased thickness of the cortex in this area could indicate that the divers are better at perceiving movements performed by others. Learning from observing others is crucial for divers – it's how they get better – and the more experienced the divers were, the thicker their cortex was in this part of the brain.

This idea of learning by observation is a powerful one in skill acquisition – remember the mirror neurons we looked at in chapter one, which fire both when you perform an action and when you see another person performing the same action. In sport, mirror neurons and neural plasticity explain how athletes are able to learn new skills, and how they learn to anticipate the actions of their opponents.

Clowns and War

It takes surprisingly little time for your brain to start changing. Although we've been talking in terms of thousands of hours of practice over the course of several years, researchers in Germany found that the plastic brain can change shape within a matter of months when someone learns a new skill. They scanned the brains of jugglers, although they started with novices, so they didn't have to try to coax clowns away from the circus into the metal tube of the fMRI machine (I wonder how many would fit?).

First, the researchers imaged the brains of 24 people, and then gave half of them three months to learn how to juggle a classic three-ball cascade. After the three months were up, they scanned their brains again and found the tell-tale expansion in grey matter volume when compared to a group that had not learnt to juggle. After another three months with no more juggling – no flaming batons or flying scimitars here – their grey matter volume had started to decline again.

So, not only does the brain act like a muscle by growing bigger in certain areas when you give it a good workout, it also seems to shrink when you neglect those skills. Of course, it's not quite as simple as that. To understand what's going on when certain areas of the brain expand or contract, we need to dig a little deeper.

Although the brain might seem from a distance to have the kind of wiring plan you would get if you hired a mad scientist to do your Christmas decorations, it's actually very logical. In chapter one, we looked at how the visual processing areas are organised topographically – the brain areas that process what you see are arranged in a grid, like a map of the world. An object in the top right-hand corner of your visual field will be processed in an area directly adjacent to the one that processes an object in the middle right of your visual field.

It turns out that other areas of the brain, including the primary motor cortex, are organised in a very similar way. If you prod one part of the brain with an electrode, you can make that person's little finger twitch.

Move along a bit and prod them again, and it will be the next finger along on the same hand. A Canadian physician called Wilder Penfield was the first person to map out how these brain areas are organised.

In the 1940s and 1950s, he pioneered a treatment for severe epilepsy known as the Montreal Procedure. This involved destroying neurons in the areas of the brain where the seizure originated. In order to find these areas, he used electrodes to stimulate different parts of the patient's brain while they were conscious (under only local anaesthetic) and see how they responded. This technique is still in use today – in certain cases brain surgeons use it when removing tumours to make sure their tools don't stray into any important areas – and there are videos online of patients speaking, singing or even playing the guitar while being operated on.

A side effect of this technique was that Penfield had the opportunity to become one of the first physicians to observe which areas of the brain connected up to which body parts. He created maps of the sensory and motor cortices of the brain, called the cortical homunculus (see diagram below), showing not only their layout, but also the relative sizes of their 'receptive fields'.

The easiest way to demonstrate the concept of a receptive field is with a little experiment. Find a trusting friend, ask them to shut their eyes and prod them somewhere on the hand with two fingers spaced an inch apart. Ask them to tell you how many fingers you just touched them with. Try again with just one finger, or with three. Alternate between them, and they should be able to get the right answer most of the time. Try altering the distance between your fingers – the closer you bring them together, the harder it will be for your friend to tell whether there's one point of contact or two. Try to find the point at which they can no longer tell the difference between one finger and two fingers touching them, if you can. That's the size of their receptive field for touch in their hand.

Next, try the same thing again, but somewhere else on their body – the upper arm or back, for example. They should find it much harder to tell how many points of contact there are over smaller distances. These areas are less sensitive than the hand, because their receptive fields are much bigger.

In your visual cortex, the centre of your retina is processed by a much larger area of your brain than the periphery, like the enlarged centre of a city street map. This is the tactile equivalent. Your fingertips connect to a much larger area of your brain than a fingertip-sized part of your back, and this is why you have much more sensitivity in your fingers.

The same applies for the motor cortex. The reason that you can probably move your fingers with a greater degree of control and precision than your toes is because your fingers are controlled by a much larger portion of your brain, as you can see in this frankly quite terrifying map of the motor homunculus, which has gone pretty much unchanged since Penfield's day.

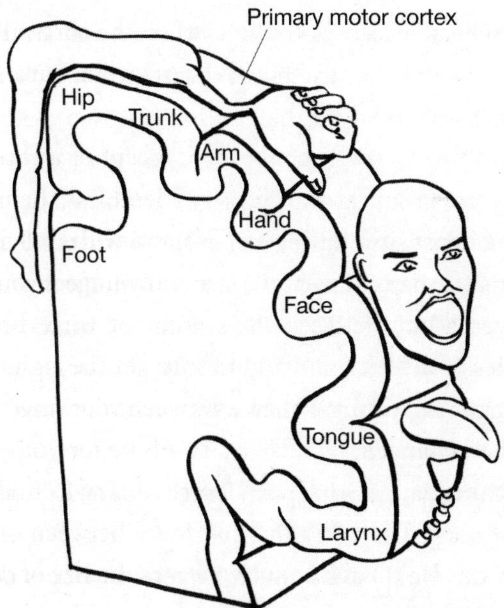

These cortical maps are not fixed. They overlap, and they can expand and contract with practice, thanks to neural plasticity.

Another study of violinists was one of the first to demonstrate that experts' brains do indeed have a different layout, altered by hours of practice. Fortunately, technology has moved on since Penfield's day, so there was no prodding the virtuosos with electrodes while they played.

Instead, the researchers used a technique called transcranial magnetic stimulation (TMS). This involves passing a coil with an electric current running through it over the skull; the magnetic field created can induce or disrupt the firing of neurons. If you pass it over the motor cortex, you can get a very similar effect to prodding it with an electrode, and by combining this with an fMRI scan, you can work out exactly which areas of the brain control which muscles in the body.

In this study the researchers were particularly interested in the muscles of the left hand. In violinists, this is the one that presses down on the strings and controls whether you get haunting melodies or screeching agony. Experts' movements have to be quick, firm and precise.

The researchers, based both in Germany and in Birmingham, Alabama, discovered that the brain area that controlled the fingers of the violinists' left hand was bigger than the same area in a control group. Meanwhile, the cortical maps for the right hand were the same size as the control group, as was the area controlling the thumb of the left hand, which just sits on the neck of the violin while playing.

Years of practice had changed the structure of the musicians' brains. There was even a link between the amount of brain reorganisation for the muscles of the left hand and the age at which each subject had started playing – the younger they were when they started, the more their brains had changed.

The same thing happens in sport. Roger Federer's racket may not be quite as finely crafted as a Stradivarius, but years of using it have still shaped his brain. He'll have a much bigger area of his brain devoted to the hand muscles than an amateur tennis player.

In 2013, in response to a slump in form, Federer made the decision to switch from a racket with a surface area of 90 square inches to one with a surface area of 100 square inches, in line with most other elite male tennis players. 'Rackets are the most important thing for a tennis player,' said former tennis pro Darren Cahill, in a *New York Times* article about Federer's switch. 'Understanding it. Knowing it. Trusting it. It's part of your family. Those stories of people putting their rackets on their bed and sleeping with them, it's what we live with. We see more of our rackets than we do of anybody else in our lives.'

Spending so much time using a tool like a tennis racket will change the brain. A group of Australian scientists looked at the cortical representations of the hand muscles in five elite badminton players, and found that the athletes had larger cortical maps for these areas than social players and those who had never played any form of racket sport.

Increasing the area of the brain that is connected to a particular muscle increases the sensitivity with which it can be consciously controlled. Some people find it tricky to move their ring fingers without their little fingers twitching as well, but pianists or guitarists can usually manage it more easily. Equally, if you were to bind two of your fingers together for a while, so that they could only move simultaneously, when you took the binding off you would find it difficult to move them separately for a while because your brain will have reorganised itself.

Changing tools can also require the brain to adjust and change. When Federer switched rackets, there will have been a period of cortical reorganisation. When Rory McIlroy signed his multimillion-dollar deal with Nike, he switched clubs, balls and everything almost overnight, and his game tanked. It took him a while to get back to the level he was at before, and it could be argued that this was due to the area of his brain that represents the relevant muscles having to make tiny readjustments to reorganise itself for the minute changes in club shape and weight.

These changes can start to happen remarkably quickly. The size of these areas is not set in stone, and adjacent areas run into each other and overlap. When I speak to Billy Morgan, he's in recovery from a serious operation on the anterior cruciate ligament in his knee. He's fidgety, itching to get active again, but he's still not allowed to run or jump yet. 'I find it so hard to hold myself back,' he says. 'I'm not supposed to skateboard at all, but if I'm going down the road to my friend's house . . . I'll drive myself crazy if I just sit in the gym doing leg presses.'

He'll be out for six months and, when he gets out on to the slopes for the first time (after some 'next-level rehab'), he won't be able immediately to do all of the things he could do before. This rusty feeling athletes get when coming back from injury is because the brain is fluid; when they're not used the neural connections start to atrophy, just like muscles. When Morgan first started his career, he would take six-month breaks in between ski seasons to work, and he would feel rusty for a few days, but this time it will take longer because he's operating at a more complex level. 'I need all the tricks that I've learnt back consistently, and that's a problem,' he says. 'A lot of the time you get a few tricks back but you're just fighting the landing on one trick for ages. I need to go away and quickly identify which tricks I need to sort out and get back into training.'

There's a territorial war going on in Morgan's head. If you break your leg and can't use it for a while, the part of the brain that controls it will get invaded by adjacent areas. Studies of amputees have found that when they lose a limb, the brain areas adjacent expand into the area. Neural resources are allocated by a bit of a free-for-all, governed by the general principle of 'use it or lose it' – like overlapping games of cricket in a crowded public park.

Strikers and Sea Slugs

When Manchester United won the treble in 1999, they owed a lot to one of the greatest strike partnerships of the modern era. Andy Cole and Dwight Yorke scored 53 goals between them that season, and seemed to have a telepathic relationship off the pitch, and what Rob Smyth in the *Guardian* calls 'the sort of instant chemistry usually reserved for slushy rom-coms'. The duo had started only one game together for United when Cole was brought into the side for a league game against Southampton in October 1998. Eleven minutes in, he picked up the ball on the left-hand side and crossed for Yorke at the near post. The Tobagonian striker scuffed his finish rather, but it crept in, and they spent the rest of the season terrorising defences together.

They were fast friends off the pitch too. 'Coley took time out to show me where to live, showed me all the places to go,' said Yorke in an interview 15 years later. 'He even invited me to the family home and fed me! I was pretty much on my own up in Manchester, but he looked after me. So when we got that opportunity to play, I think that helped. It was that bond we had.'

Would Cole and Yorke have scored quite as many goals together if they didn't get on? Or perhaps if that first, scuffed shot from Yorke had trickled wide instead of into the net, the game against Southampton wouldn't have been the start of a beautiful friendship. I mention this because it illustrates one of the key principles of neural plasticity. Because our thoughts and memories are made up of the connections between billions of neurons, changing them requires changing the strength of the connections between individual neurons.

Each neuron resembles an uprooted tree. The roots of the tree, called dendrites, are long and thin; they collect signals from other neurons. At the opposite end of each neuron is the axon, which is longer and thicker, and branches out at the top to pass signals on to other neurons. Between the axon of one neuron and the dendrite of the next, there's a gap called a synapse. This is a gap that electrical impulses can't cross, and so, when a neuron fires, it releases neurotransmitters – chemical messengers that float across the gap to pass the message on to the next neuron and trigger it to fire.

When one neuron causes another one to fire, or when two neurons fire in close succession, the connection between them becomes strengthened due to chemical changes at the synapses. It's a simple rule: neurons that fire together wire together.

This idea is an old one. It was first suggested by Sigmund Freud, but is now known as Hebb's Law, after being outlined in Donald Hebb's 1949 book *The Organisation of Behaviour.* Its precise chemical workings weren't pinned down until the 1960s, when neuropsychiatrist Eric Kandel started working with a giant marine slug called *Aplysia californica.* These sea slugs are unique because they have only around 20,000 neurons, and their neurons are unusually large and translucent, which allows them to be easily studied. By isolating a single neural circuit within the sea slug, Kandel was able to identify the changes that happen at the synapses when memories are made.

Communication between neurons is controlled by neurotransmitters, which are released from one neuron and travel across the synapse where they bind with receptors on the next neuron, triggering it to fire.

When two neurons fire together, their connection is strengthened. A gene is activated which changes the structure of the neurons on both sides of the synapse: the first one changes so that it will release more neurotransmitters in future, and the second one develops more receptors for those neurotransmitters to bind to. Opening one door causes more to be built. One study by Kandel and colleagues found that the number of receptors in a single neuron could more than double during this process.

That is the basic mechanism of learning and memory. When you experience something or perform an action, your neurons fire in sequence, each one triggering those around it. The very act of them firing together strengthens the connections between them, as neurotransmitters are released, receptors are grown and new synaptic connections are built. That's how cortical maps change shape. But that's not the only change. There are tales from the training field from every sport about players who went the extra mile. At Manchester United, David Beckham emerged from a culture of staying behind after training to practise free kicks, and made himself one of the greatest strikers of a dead ball in the history of football. Right-handed snooker great Ronnie O'Sullivan practised with his left hand to the point where he is able to use it in matchplay situations.

Even after you've mastered a skill, practice can be beneficial. It makes the brain more efficient. Think of employees in a job they've been doing for years. They know the demands of the task well, so they're very good at it, and they're also able to complete their work to the same standard as before but without having to put in as much effort. The same thing happens with neurons in the brain.

When you learn a new skill, your cortical map for the area of the body you're using expands, but eventually you need fewer neurons and less energy to do the same job because you learn to use your muscles more efficiently. You can observe the effects of this increased neural efficiency in the best sportspeople. Watch Lionel Messi control a pass and look at his economy of movement, the lightness of his touch, compared to a League 2 player. Similarly, observe the way a fielder's body moves as they throw the ball, the fluidity of the action, compared to your own efforts, or the way Roger Federer's forehand arm seems to float through the air when he plays a perfectly judged winner.

Neymar was one of the biggest names in world football even before he made his multimillion-euro transfer from Brazilian club Santos to join Messi at Barcelona. He was the son of a footballer, grew up playing futsal and street football, and was spotted by Santos and signed up at the age of just 11, so it's fair to say he'd got his 10,000 hours of practice in pretty early on.

In 2014, researchers in Japan got the chance to examine how much more efficient all that practice had made Neymar's brain. They scanned him in an fMRI machine while he rotated his right ankle clockwise or anti-clockwise every few seconds. Compared to three other professional footballers, two top swimmers and an amateur footballer who did the same task, they found that the brain activity during this task was smaller in the footballers than in the swimmers, smaller in the professional footballers than the amateurs, and smallest of all in Neymar's brain.

The researchers believe this unique pattern of brain activity comes from Neymar's years of practice of playing barefoot with nearly 50 different types of ball. His brain has changed. The connections between neurons have been strengthened. The area of the brain that controls his feet has grown bigger, but has also become more efficient.

We might call this muscle memory in layman's terms, and this increasing neural efficiency is just one part of it. The other aspect involves speeding things up, with the help of a fatty substance called myelin – the brain's white matter.

Auto(Maticity)Bahn

Why do athletes peak at a certain age? Yes, their bodies start to rebel after years of being pushed to the limit, but their mental skills start to deteriorate too. They can't react as quickly to things as they used to, and there's only so long that their increased experience can offset this loss of basic speed.

A neuron is like an electrical wire. Insulating a wire means the current within will flow faster and more efficiently. Myelin is the body's electrical insulation. Changes at the synapses hold the key to learning, but myelin controls the manifestation of that learning. Myelin wraps around neurons, like insulation around a copper wire. It keeps the signals in, so they can travel faster, with less signal loss. 'Myelin quietly transforms narrow alleys into broad, lightning-fast super-highways,' writes Daniel Coyle in *The Talent Code*. 'Neural traffic that once trundled along at two miles an hour can, with myelin's help, accelerate to two hundred miles an hour.'

Myelinating a neural pathway is like upgrading it from dial-up to broadband. Combined with a decrease in the gap required before the neuron can send another signal, these changes lead to a 3,000-fold increase in processing capacity. As we've seen, a crucial thing that separates athletes from the rest of us is their ability to pick up perceptual cues ahead of time, and to make decisions quickly and accurately. Speed is of the essence, and myelin is the essence of speed.

When a neuron fires, not only does it strengthen the connection to the neurons around it, it also attracts the attention of cells called oligodendrocytes, which resemble *Space Invaders* in brain images, glowing an eerie green. They build myelin, squeezing out a layer of coating that wraps itself precisely around the neuron in an ongoing process that can take relative aeons in the brain's super-fast timescales.

'It's one of the most intricate and exquisite cell-to-cell processes there is,' says Dr Douglas Fields in *The Talent Code*. 'And it's slow. Each one of these wraps can go around the nerve fibre forty or fifty times, and can take days or weeks. Imagine doing that to an entire neuron, then an entire circuit with thousands of nerves. It would be like insulating a transatlantic cable.'

No wonder, then, that it takes experts 10,000 hours to develop their skills. Not only do they have to create the neural pathways – the long-term memories of the knowledge they need to perform – they also need to build up their bandwidth, the myelin coating around the neurons which will grant them speed and efficiency. 'Skill is a cellular insulation that wraps neural circuits and that grows in response to certain signals,' writes Coyle, repeatedly.

But, as we'll discover in Part Two, there could be shortcuts to skill, ways of speeding up the process of neural plasticity. By optimising the signals we send the brain through training, we can maximise neural plasticity, speed up the development of myelin and break the 10,000-hour rule.

Billy Morgan is testament to the fact that it can be done. He didn't actually get to practise on snow until just nine years ago. 'I went skiing with my school – my mate wanted to try it and he dragged me along to the dry slope in Southampton. I didn't really want to go,' he says, but he caught the bug quickly. 'We were just addicted for two years. I didn't go on snow until I was 17.'

He came 10th at the Olympics in 2012, aged 23, despite having many thousands of hours less experience of actual snowboarding than the other competitors. But, crucially, he had managed to very efficiently train his aerial awareness – one of the key attributes for success in modern slopestyle snowboarding. Morgan started out as a gymnast. There was even a possibility of him joining a German circus at 17 ('I might still do it,' he jokes).

'I believe that the more time you spend in the air, the more comfortable you'll be and the more you'll be able to wriggle out of situations when it does go wrong,' he tells me. 'I already had that from being an acrobat when I was younger. I started gymnastics when I was, like, four years old. I was a gymnast until I was about eight and an acrobat until I was 14 and it was quite religious – every day after school, every Saturday.'

A lot of snowboarders now use the trampoline to improve their aerial ability, but Morgan had a massive head start. 'Snowboarding has become such an aerial-based sport, and the basic skills can be learnt elsewhere,' he says. 'You can do more on a trampoline – you get heaps more time in the air. It was my life, it was all I did, and I owe it all to that really, for just pounding aerial awareness into my head all the time. Without realising it, it was the conditioning that pretty much set me up to be a snowboarder.'

Morgan is able to compete with and beat people with many more years of snowboarding experience than he has because he unknowingly zeroed in on one of the key mental attributes required for his sport, and found a way to train it much more efficiently than he would have been able to on the slopes.

The content and quality of training are important. The original 10,000-hour rule specifies 'deliberate practice' – there's no point staying within your comfort zone. Thousands of hours of practising the same trick won't make you an expert in anything except that trick.

Deliberate practice is self-critical and it keeps you on the edge of your abilities, in the sweet spot where new neural connections can be made and strengthened, and the right pathways can be streamlined. 'Experiences where you're forced to slow down, make errors, and correct them – as you would if you were walking up an ice-covered hill, slipping and stumbling as you go – end up making you swift and graceful without your realising it,' writes Coyle. Your brain changes no matter what you do, but in adults it's usually only when you pay close attention to something that those changes last.

The way practice is structured can also influence neural plasticity. Massed practice has been found to increase the degree of change within the brain. The best example of this is perhaps immersion in a foreign language. A month in rural France could improve your language skills more than years of weekly lessons, because you'll be forced out of your comfort zone and into the sweet spot for learning.

Professional athletes are already immersed in their training environment, of course, but the amateur athlete could benefit from this. Early in his career, Morgan would work for six months and then spend six months snowboarding – a perfect example of massed practice. He likely improved and changed his brain more quickly than he would have if he'd spread out his time between working and snowboarding more evenly.

The brain also learns more quickly when we've been active. Exercise is one of the best catalysts for plasticity. It's hard to underestimate how powerful an effect exercise can have on our brains. It has been linked with a better ability to deal with stress, lower levels of anxiety and depression, and a wide range of improvements in learning and memory.

The effect of exercise on plasticity comes from a surge in a protein called brain-derived neurotrophic factor (BDNF). It makes neurons grow, and kick-starts synaptic plasticity. 'Early on, researchers found that if they sprinkled BDNF onto neurons in a petri dish, the cells automatically sprouted new branches, producing the same structural growth required for learning, and causing me to think of BDNF as Miracle-Gro for the brain,' writes Dr John Ratey in *Spark!*, a book which dives into the link between physical activity and learning much more deeply. Increased levels of BDNF have been found after exercise not only in the areas associated with movement, but also in the hippocampus, which is involved in the formation of new memories.

For athletes, structuring training sessions so that any tactical aspects come at the end, after the plasticity boost provided by physical exertion, could help the lessons stick.

Building a reward system into practice can also help. The neurotransmitter dopamine has a key role to play here. It is released whenever we receive a reward, whether that's in real life or in a virtual setting. Smartphone games are expertly designed to manipulate the dopamine system, feeding people with just enough reward (in the form of points, gold coins to spend, or new outfits for their character) to keep them playing.

Dopamine has also been found to enhance plasticity, so the best training methods feature an in-built reward system that not only encourages us to keep practising, but also helps the brain consolidate what we've learnt.

In the next chapter we'll look at how cutting-edge training methods and cognitive tools are taking advantage of what we now know about neural plasticity to enhance the formation of neural pathways and speed up myelin formation. But there may be other ways to achieve the same goal.

Scientists are delving deep into the foundations of our neural architecture and uncovering potentially sinister ways of maximising and accelerating neural plasticity which could change sport, and everything else, forever.

World War Lance

'You have a blank period during World War I. Then a blank period during World War II. And then one during World War Lance.'

That's disgraced former cyclist Lance Armstrong discussing the gap in the list of Tour de France winners left by his seven titles being struck from the records. It's just one example of the scourge of doping on elite sport. Cyclists and sprinters in particular are dogged by allegations and questions about performance-enhancing drugs, even if they've never failed a test.

Up until now, the bulk of the controversy has been directed at what I like to call 'output sports', where speed, strength or stamina hold more weight than high-speed decision-making. But a new storm could soon engulf a whole different range of sporting pursuits – neural doping could be elite sport's next big crisis.

When you learn something new, neural plasticity works by altering the number of neurotransmitters and receptors at the synapses to make it easier for one neuron to transmit a message to its neighbours (this is how cells that fire together wire together). But there's another way of making it easier for that message to be sent – by altering the overall balance of neurotransmitters within the brain. Recreational and medicinal drugs already take advantage of this, for example by increasing the amount of dopamine, the neurotransmitter that's released when we score a goal or complete a level on Candy Crush.

The drug Ritalin is often prescribed (some would argue too often) to disruptive children. It works by increasing the activity of dopamine within the brain, and thereby increasing focus levels. It has also been found to increase synaptic plasticity. Other drugs, such as dextro-amphetamines, have been shown to enhance memory formation in stroke patients.

There are already examples of university students taking such medication while revising for their finals, and it's possible that the same drugs could increase plasticity in athletes as well, making it easier for them to learn and improve their skills and decision-making. One study of amateur triathletes in Germany found that 15.1 per cent of them had taken substances to enhance their cognitive performance within the last year.

Some of the substances that can enhance neural plasticity are stimulants that are already on the World Anti-Doping Agency's banned list. Other methods may be harder to detect.

One of the issues when banned athletes return to their sport after drugs violations is the question of whether they're still reaping the rewards of previous illegal activities. It's hard to prove, and could be even harder when it comes to the brain. Neuroscientists at Johns Hopkins University in Baltimore conducted an experiment in which they asked volunteers to move a cursor around a screen by squeezing a sensor between their thumb and index finger. They had to move the cursor between a series of targets as quickly as possible without overshooting, learning to use the right amount of force over time. They trained for 45 minutes a day for five days, and were making far fewer errors by the end of the training.

Another group did the same learning task, but with a battery connected to their heads, which sent a current through the brain's motor cortex (which controls movement). This group learnt better; they moved the cursor faster and made fewer errors than the control group, and they retained their superior performance three months later. Other research, with stroke patients, has found that stimulating the motor cortex with TMS (transcranial magnetic stimulation) can improve their movements.

'Such interventions may with some likelihood be part of the treatment repertoire offered by future neuro-rehabilitation units for the benefit of disabled people and – who knows – may also be found in the gym of athletes training for the Olympics or alternatively on the list of illegitimate doping remedies,' writes Professor Jens Bo Nielsen, who worked on similar research at the University of Copenhagen.

When you're young, your brain is a sponge, soaking up as much information as it can and changing in response to stimuli even if you're not paying attention. This is what neuroscientists call a 'critical period', a time during development when the brain's plasticity is in overdrive. During critical periods, the brain is extra malleable and new cortical maps are made with ease.

Critical periods explain why it's easier to learn a language when you're younger, and why you're less likely to speak it with an accent if you do. They explain how we can go from knowing pretty much nothing when we're born to being able to walk, speak and understand abstract concepts by the time we're a few years old.

The nucleus basalis is a group of neurons deep in the brain involved in focusing our attention. During a critical period, it goes into overdrive, allowing learning to take place almost effortlessly from birth until around the age of 10 or 11. It's switched on and off by a massive release of BDNF – the same plasticity-boosting brain protein released during exercise.

Once the nucleus basalis is switched off, the critical period is over, and long-term changes to the brain only take place when something important happens, or when we make an effort to pay attention. It's why babies can pick up the rules of language and grammar effortlessly, but learning them as an adult takes hours of rote study and staring at verb tables.

If we could find the key to unlocking critical periods, it would spark a revolution, not just in sport but in all areas of skill acquisition and expertise. It may just be possible.

Neuroplasticity pioneers Michael Kilgard and Michael Merzenich were able to train newborn rats – still in their critical period – to differentiate between musical notes just by playing them repeatedly. At first, their auditory cortex could only differentiate between high and low notes, but over time it developed specific areas that would fire when exposed to a C#, for example.

By inserting micro-electrodes into the nucleus basalis of *adult* rats, Merzenich and Kilgard were able to switch the critical period back on. The rats effortlessly developed brain maps when played the tones, just like newborn rats who were still in their critical period. The researchers had reopened the window for rapid learning.

Techniques like this, and others with potential such as injecting BDNF directly into the brain, are years or decades away from being used in humans, and obviously there are ethical concerns to be grappled with. But, now more than ever, sport is operating on the fringes of science and technology. Where there is an advantage to be gained on the field, you can bet that somewhere, someone is investing the money to chisel it out. There is an awakening going on among coaches from basketball to football and beyond.

In Part One, we've learnt how neural plasticity helps athletes' brains become uniquely specialised for anticipation and high-speed decision-making. In Part Two, we'll meet some of the people who are using our growing knowledge of the brain to push the boundaries of performance and reveal some tips that could help your own sporting endeavours.

Try this at home:

BOOST YOUR BRAIN'S LEARNING POWER

Massed practice

If you've been struggling to learn a new skill, whether it's a sport or a language, the research suggests that you might be better off diving right into it for an extended period of time, rather than spreading out your efforts over the course of weekly lessons. Early on in his career, slopestyle snowboarder Billy Morgan would work for six months and then spend six months snowboarding – his brain would have changed more quickly than it would have if he'd spread out his snowboarding more evenly.

The power of exercise

Exercising boosts the levels of a brain protein called BDNF, which has been found to massively increase the rate at which neurons grow new branches. In other words, exercising can make you better at learning and remembering new skills and information. Try studying after exercise instead of before, and you could take advantage of this in-built learning boost.

Part Two

THE BRAIN-TRAINING EXPLOSION

CHAPTER FOUR

BREAKING THE 10,000-HOUR RULE

Mustafa Amini stands, ready. Keeping on his toes, the Borussia Dortmund player waits for the signal. It comes from behind him – an unnatural noise like a car being remotely unlocked, and a flash of red light. Amini spins towards the sound as a football flies towards him. He traps the ball with his right foot, and then with a second touch sends it neatly through a hole in the opposite wall that has been marked out by green lights.

Amini is inside the Footbonaut. As we'll discover in this chapter, it's just one of the innovative ways in which sports teams are using new technology to train brains as well as bodies.

The Footbonaut has been installed at German clubs Borussia Dortmund and TSG Hoffenheim, and by a handful of other football teams and academies around the world. It is a square of Astroturf, 14 metres by 14 metres (46 feet by 46 feet), with a white circle painted in the middle, and four walls that are divided up by squares into a total of 64 targets. It's like standing inside the wooden frame of a house before the plasterboard goes up.

There are ball-firing machines on each wall of the room, eight in total. The player stands in the middle of the room; there's a warning noise and a flash of red light, and a football is fired at him from an unpredictable direction and at an unpredictable speed – anything up to 60 miles an hour. As the ball is released, a second noise sounds and a flash of green light illuminates one of the 64 target gates. The player has to control the ball and pass it through the target as quickly as possible. The sounds and flashing lights combine to make the whole experience seem like a mix between *Tron* and Nike's 'The Cage' advertising campaign from the mid-2000s.

Dystopian science-fiction overtones aside, the players are unanimous in their support for the Footbonaut, which is supposed to help improve passing accuracy and can also send data about the player's performance to a tablet computer where it can be analysed by a coach. 'The facility is great,' said Amini, a 23-year-old Australian who was playing in Dortmund's B team at the time. 'The repetition of ball you get helps your technique and your vision, and helps you open up and look for the target.'

World Cup winner Mario Gotze agrees. When the Footbonaut was first introduced at Dortmund in 2012, he loved it so much he would play on it long into the night. 'I can only recommend it,' he said at the time. 'It's something amazing. It's a good opportunity to improve yourself technically and get better vision, a better passing game. It gives a lot of opportunities to improve and work on your weak points. I think it is a good way to practise.' Gotze, now at Bayern Munich, scored the winning goal in the 2014 World Cup final deep into extra time – a cross from the left at an awkward height, which he chested down and volleyed past the Argentinian keeper. A Footbonaut goal.

In August 2015, I went to Hoffenheim to try out the Footbonaut for myself, and find out how the club are using it alongside other tools to give their players the edge in the Bundesliga. Hoffenheim is an unusual place for a top-flight football club; it's no more than a village really, but its football team was boosted by a large injection of cash from local software billionaire Dietmar Hopp. The co-founder of SAP had played youth football at the club, who were in the fifth tier of German football when he first took an interest around 15 years ago. They've flown up through the divisions since, and now boast a €100m, 30,000-seater stadium and some of the best training facilities money can buy. They don't look that high-tech from the outside, however. It's all very rural in the German countryside, and I have to overtake a tractor towards the end of my journey from the airport to the club's base in a converted castle in Zuzenhausen, a nearby village.

Jan Mayer is waiting for me inside. Hoffenheim's sports psychologist has the receding hairline and thick-framed glasses of a career academic. He has been working in football for 15 years, and has written several books on the subjects of coaching and sport psychology. Inside the castle, the club's offices feel more like a medical clinic, all clean white corridors and keypad entry systems. The Footbonaut is housed in a separate, hangar-like construction at the end of a gravel drive. It cost more than €2m to build. 'Welcome to my baby,' Mayer laughs, as he buzzes us in and switches on the lights. 'Would you like to have a go?'

It is genuinely one of the most entertaining things I have ever done. Mayer picks up an iPad and selects the desired speed, height and number of incoming passes, and the difficulty of targets (there are two rows, but I'm on easy mode and just using the bottom layer), while I stand in the centre of the machine inside the white circle. I can see the gates – about two feet by two feet– arranged in a grid around the room in rows and columns. But where are the ball machines?

I get my answer as Mayer taps 'start' on the iPad. There's a theatrical whoosh, like a spaceship door opening, and panels at around head height slide open, revealing my robotic teammates. Two sounds play. The first comes from the machine that is going to be releasing the ball, the second quickly afterwards, from the direction of the target. The first ball comes at a decent pace, and I focus on controlling it neatly, which I manage to do. Unfortunately, I've completely failed to clock where I'm supposed to be passing it to, so there's an awkward spin as I look around, which isn't going to do wonders for my score. The Footbonaut measures your time as well as your accuracy.

A couple more passes go by before I figure out that I need to glance around to locate the target before the ball gets to me, so I don't take forever searching for it after I've controlled the ball. The noise and setting create a strange sense of urgency – I'm definitely leaning towards speed more than accuracy. Six passes received and (eventually) dispatched, and it's game over – which the machine announces in a robotic voice that reminds me so much of ITV's game show *The Cube* that it actually makes me laugh out loud. Fifteen minutes later, and perspiring slightly after two more turns and 30 more passes received, I'm in Mayer's office, where he talks me through some of the science around the Footbonaut.

Despite the eye-catching and futuristic dressing, the thought process behind the machine is quite straightforward. Legendary coach Bill Shankly won three first division titles with Liverpool in the 1960s and 1970s using similar training techniques. 'We brought out the training boards,' Shankly said. 'They would be set up about 15 yards apart and would keep the ball in play and keep the players on the move all the time. If the ball beat the goalkeeper, it would hit a board and be back in play again. We also had a "sweat box", using boards like the walls of a house, with the players playing the ball off the wall on to the next. The ball was played against the board, you controlled it, turned around, and took it again.'

Nowadays we have a much better idea of why these training techniques yield results. As well as keeping the muscles strong and the body in shape, they also train the brain. The key to both the Footbonaut and the 'sweat box' is repetition – it allows players to receive and make many more passes than they would during an ordinary training session, but in the same amount of time. The Footbonaut's creator, Berlin-based designer Christian Guttler, claims that in just 15 minutes in his machine a player can receive and make as many passes as they would in a week of normal football training.

A number of less expensive pieces of training equipment have sprung up that adhere to this principle of making training more efficient. One is SenseBall, favoured by pioneering Belgian coach Michel Bruyninckx, who we'll meet later. This is essentially a football inside a small net: a young player holds the net in one hand and practises kicking the ball with different parts of his feet as it bounces back to him after each touch. It's not a million miles away from kicking a ball against a wall in your garden, except without the risk of smashed windows.

Another is called Topspin Pro. This £99 contraption consists of a tennis ball mounted on a fixed wire and surrounded by a mesh screen. The idea is to hit the tennis ball to make it spin as much as possible but without hitting the screen, thereby training the exact motion required to hit a shot with topspin but without the need for a partner to play against.

Efficiency and richness of training are thought to be two of the reasons why Brazil has produced so many great footballers over the years. Futsal, a favoured variant of the game played on a small pitch with a small, heavy ball, gives players many more touches than they'd get in a traditional game – six times as many according to one study. 'Futsal makes you think fast and play fast,' Brazilian legend Pele has said. 'You try things, it makes you dribble. It makes you a better player.'

Football has changed a bit since Pele's day (you wouldn't see him scoring a thousand goals now), and futsal alone may not be enough to give players the edge they need in the modern game. According to research that Mayer tells me about, passing is now 35 per cent quicker and more accurate than it was at the 1966 World Cup. The rate of change seems to be increasing, as indicated by the German FA's analysis of its men's national team at the 2006 World Cup, where they came third, and the 2014 World Cup, which they won. Average ball contact time for their team across the tournament fell from 2.9 seconds in 2006 to just 0.9 seconds in 2014 – the German players were holding on to the ball for less time, and making decisions more quickly.

Midfielder Bastian Schweinsteiger was part of both of those squads. 'In elite soccer, it is often minor details, virtually imperceptible from outside, that decide who wins and loses,' he said in an interview with *Kicker* magazine. 'The key is to think and act rapidly. I find it fascinating to master these minor details.'

'In 10 years' time, this game is going to be three times faster,' Mayer tells me. 'Being faster is not only about muscles or about tactics – it's in the head of course.'

Train Above The Neck

The GlaxoSmithKline Human Performance Lab (HPL) doesn't look much like the future of anything, from the outside. It's in a squat industrial unit in Brentford, Middlesex, across the M4 from the pharmaceutical company's towering headquarters. Inside, though, behind a wall that slides open at the touch of a button, it's a state-of-the-art sports science lab.

There are treadmills, immersion pools, weight machines and a range of other tools that researchers are using to test the capabilities of elite athletes, and how these might change with different types of nutrition or hydration. As well as sweat and sugar, the scientists here are also interested in the mental side of sport. Behind frosted glass doors etched with the word 'Cognition', the HPL's chief neuroscientist, Dr Barry O'Neill, shows me some of the training tools his team have been developing in conjunction with an American company called Axon Sports.

Axon Sports' equipment has been installed by a number of professional and college teams across the United States and elsewhere. 'We want to be able to provide athletes with ways to make the number of decisions you would make in a season over the course of two weeks,' the company's president, Jason Sada, tells me. Their mantra is 'train above the neck', and they have a range of different computer and touch-screen-based tools, each adapted to the specific needs of a particular position in a particular sport.

We've seen how athletes' brains are adapted to make high-speed decisions through thousands of hours of practice, and Axon Sports are among those trying to tap into, train and potentially shorten that process. 'Fundamentally, we believe that in the vast majority of sports the dominating function for an athlete's success or failure is built around high-speed decision-making,' says Sada. 'There's a huge requirement on the athlete's cognitive system to not only make accurate decisions but to make them incredibly fast. We always use the analogy that 100 per cent accuracy that's always late is inherently going to lead to failure. If you identify the things properly but you see them too late you're not able to capitalise on the identification.'

A typical example of one of Axon Sports' training tools involves baseball, and helps hitters train their anticipation skills. By exposing them to many more pitches than they would see in regular practice, the company's software helps players learn the advance cues they need to react quickly.

The athlete stands in front of a large touch screen, with arms raised as if holding a bat ready to swing. A video of a pitcher is shown in front of him but it stops at the moment the ball is about to be released, and the hitter has to identify what kind of pitch is coming, or the location of where the ball is going, by tapping one of several options presented on the screen. It's like some of those early occlusion experiments, but turned into a game instead of a test. The hitter can see a new pitch every few seconds, without wearing out the body or risking injury. 'We can train the athlete without the odometer running,' says Sada.

At the HPL, O'Neill and his team have been tweaking Axon Sports' tools for use in football, rugby and cricket. The principle is the same, but for rugby and football developing the tools is more challenging because they are what O'Neill calls 'open loop' sports: outside of set pieces, any player could be pretty much anywhere on the pitch and anything can happen. In contrast, American football, baseball and cricket are 'closed loop' sports – the action resets after each play.

For rugby, O'Neill shows me two examples, one offensive and one defensive, selecting the options he wants from a slickly designed interface on a wall-mounted screen. 'Obviously we wouldn't call them "offense" and "de-fense" in the UK, but we haven't got round to changing that yet,' he says, laughing, when those two menu items come up.

O'Neill's team have worked in conjunction with local rugby clubs in west London to film sequences that provide the raw training material. 'In order to isolate the cognitive skills that are crucial to different sports and positions we need to work with people who know the sports,' he says. 'So you can either do it through scripted shoots where you get people to set up the scenarios or you can use game footage and stop it at particular points.'

A video clip shows a rugby player running towards the camera with the ball tucked under his arm. At the end of the clip, just before he reaches the viewer, two arrows appear, and the user has to tap the direction they think the player is going to go – left or right. O'Neill taps away to demonstrate how the arrow lights up green if they've got it right, and how players using the system accrue points for speed and accuracy.

For football it's slightly more complicated. The HPL are using real game footage from New England Revolution, a Major League Soccer team. A clip from a game plays out over a few seconds, and then multiple options for the player in possession appear on the screen; in this case, they are a straight pass to the left, a long ball into space, or the option to hold on to the ball and dribble either to the left or to the right. Again players have to choose what they think is the best option based on the information available.

'You can give people a volume of training that you couldn't tolerate physically,' says Professor Bruce Abernethy, the Australian whose work on occlusion paved the way for tools like these. 'All along, the intent has been not just to document that some people can predict better than others; but then the next step is to find where that critical information is, and then, having found it, try and present it in an augmented way that will speed up learning.'

'It absolutely can be a shortcut,' says Dr Peter Fadde, an instructional engineer at the University of Southern Illinois who has developed occlusion techniques to train pitch recognition in baseball. 'That's the goal of it. That's what they're really interested in – accelerated expertise. Take what would be a natural learning progression and systematise it so we get more people over that bar faster.'

Find out what experts do differently. Home in on it, and try to find a way of exposing your trainees to that stimulus, but more efficiently. This is how the 10,000-hour rule can be broken.

'What Does This Have To Do With Baseball?'

Elite teams are generally pretty reluctant to share their trade secrets, so there are few professional-level case studies out there of this kind of technology in action – but it is being used. The Boston Red Sox are known to be working with NeuroScouting, another brain-training company. Participation in iPad- and laptop-based games became compulsory for their reserve teams in 2010 – 10- or 20-minute sessions in hotels, dressing rooms or on the team bus. 'It was part of our routine because it was sort of forced on us,' outfielder Jackie Bradley Jr told the *Boston Globe*. 'It was a competitive thing because there were rankings. That's what kept it fun. If it wasn't like that, it would have been like homework.'

The games are simpler than the video-based tools currently being developed by Axon Sports. Instead of video footage, players see a virtual pitch, an animated ball coming towards them.

The Red Sox also have been using the programme for recruitment. One player, Mookie Betts, was drafted partly because he excelled at these computer-based tasks. 'I missed my lunch period because I was doing NeuroScouting,' Betts said, recalling the day a Red Sox scout came to visit him at his high school and put him through the tests. '[The scout] just said, "Do this, don't think about the results." I did what I could. It was just, like, a ball popped up, tap space bar as fast as you could. If the seams were one way, you tapped it. If it was the other way, you weren't supposed to tap it. I was getting some of them wrong. I wasn't getting frustrated, but I was like, "Dang, this is hard."'

'I was thinking, "What does this have to do with baseball?"' Betts said in another interview. 'I guess I did pretty well, since he kept on pursuing me.' He credits the software with helping him break into the major leagues. 'It gets your brain going,' he said. Betts is now considered one of the best young players in baseball.

Not all players have taken to it with quite the same level of enthusiasm. 'For the most part, guys just seem, like, every other day, "Ugh I have to do this again,"' Tampa Bay Rays outfielder Kevin Kiermaier told the *Wall Street Journal*. 'You try to get in a routine, and it's like, "Oh, you have to do neuroscience or you're going to get fined."'

Despite the reluctance of some, this kind of training has yielded tangible results on the field, according to Sada. 'We implemented the pitch-recognition and location-based assessments in training for a baseball team and every hitting category went up, every single one of them. In one case a coach saw every hitting category go up with the exception of doubles, and the reason for that was that triples had replaced the doubles.' A double in baseball is when a batter hits the ball and manages to run around to second base, a triple is when they make it round to third base.

Fadde managed a similarly striking improvement when he implemented his pitch-recognition training at Southeast Missouri State College. He used video training, and also real-world occlusion techniques including nets and screens. 'I tried having guys hold a piece of plywood so that the pitch would disappear, but the pitch would hit the plywood or it would hit the player. I finally realised that by simply having them [the batters] call out "yes" or "no", "ball" or "strike" before the pitch hits the catcher's mitt forces their recognition time into exactly the same point that you're working on with the video when you cut it off. I call it attention occlusion.'

Between 2013 and 2014, when they implemented Fadde's training, the college team's runs per game went up by 48 per cent, and the number of home runs increased by 127 per cent.

'What we've seen with this training across the board is that hitting has improved,' says Sada. 'So your home run numbers will go up, your walk to strikeout ratio will go up; all of these elements will increase because the decision-making prior to swinging the bat has improved. That's what we've seen as we've deployed this out, and it really has been pretty amazing.'

The Million-Dollar Brain

For my research project at university, I spent a summer term crudely doctoring pop songs on my laptop. I was looking for a link between the way that music and language are processed in the brain. When people hear a grammatical mistake, they display a particular pattern of brain activity, and I wanted to see whether expert musicians displayed a similar pattern when they heard musical mistakes. This involved taking a number of short clips from famous pieces of music, ranging from classical songs such as Beethoven's Fifth to modern classics like the theme tune from *Jurassic Park*, and altering certain notes so that they were played in the wrong key, or for the wrong length of time, or on the wrong instrument.

To measure the brain activity of my participants – a mixture of Grade 8 musicians and non-expert undergraduates who were paid £5 for their co-operation – I used an electroencephalogram, or EEG. This is usually what people are referring to when they talk about measuring brain waves.

It consists of a device that looks like a cross between a swimming cap, a colander and an improvised explosive device. The holes are electrodes; you put the cap on, squirt a conductive gel into each of them to connect them electrically to the scalp, plug the wires into a computer, and you can then measure the electrical activity taking place under the skull at a number of different sites. It's painless, but a little uncomfortable, as you have to remain quite still.

My friend Tom was the first person to be subjected to my musical creations, but your typical day one teething problems meant that instead of moving from track to track, he actually ended up hearing a horribly twisted version of Aqua's 'Barbie Girl' 17 times in a row. He has never been quite the same since.

Jason Sherwin laughs when I tell him about this ('How did you get ethical approval for that?!?'), because he once ran a very similar experiment with musicians, before moving on to scanning the brains of baseball players when they make decisions about incoming pitches. 'If it makes you feel any better, in the first pilot experiment we did with musicians we did "Eye of the Tiger" by Survivor,' he tells me over Skype from his office in Chicago. 'So whenever this friend of mine is driving in the car and he hears "Eye of the Tiger" he still remembers where we put the key changes in that song.'

Sherwin is in his early thirties, and his background is varied. He did his undergraduate degree in physics and music, and a masters and a doctorate in aerospace engineering. But, thanks to growing up playing baseball and watching the Chicago Cubs, he has ended up in the world of sports. He is one of the founder members of deCervo, a company that uses EEGs to scan the brains of baseball players as they make decisions about incoming pitches, taking the pitch-recognition training software one step further than the likes of Axon Sports. 'They're doing black-and-white television with rabbit-ear antennas – we're doing HD with satellite,' Sherwin boasts in one interview.

Like fMRI, EEG is not without its flaws. While it is very good at measuring the timing of events within the brain, because it is measured through the scalp it is not great at localising those events. Trying to read the brain using fMRI is a bit like following a football match on a live text blog – you get a vague, delayed idea of what is going on. EEG, on the other hand, is like standing outside the ground listening to the crowd; you'll know before anyone at home if a goal has been scored, but you'll have less idea of what has actually happened.

DeCervo's work has grown out of research at Columbia University, New York. For the last few years, armed with just a laptop and a black aluminium briefcase, Sherwin and his business partner Jordan Muraskin have been travelling up and down the country visiting baseball teams in training. They want to figure out the timing of pitch recognition in the brain.

The briefcase contains a $10,000 EEG kit from Advanced Brain Monitoring, essentially a sleeker, sexier version of the one I used for my undergraduate research project. Not that scalp gel can ever really be considered sexy. 'Players don't want to wear something that looks like a Hydra on their heads, with all these wires going everywhere,' Muraskin told sports news website SB Nation. 'They want small and sleek.'

Sherwin and Muraskin showed players different computer-generated pitches – just a green dot moving towards them against a blank background. Players were told the pitch would be a certain type, a fastball, a curveball or a slider, and they were asked to press a button only if that was actually the case.

By cross-referencing the EEG measurements with their answers, Sherwin and team were able to find out that fastballs were recognised quickest (which makes sense as they're the stock delivery, so players have more experience of them), while it took longer for curveballs to be recognised. The pitches were generally recognised when the ball was between 32 and 40 feet from the plate, in the middle third of the delivery. 'There's usually a jump [in brain activity] around 300 or 350 milliseconds, where the player really starts recognising the pitch,' said Muraskin.

Following that research, the pair carried out another study in which they combined the timing data from the EEG with an fMRI scan so that they could model exactly where this recognition-primed decision-making happens in the brain. They managed to convince college baseball players to lie in an fMRI machine while wearing an EEG cap and watching a variety of different pitches. 'We were able to link some of the aspects of how they see the ball to previous work on highly specialised structures in the brain that are used for visual object recognition,' Sherwin tells me. 'Particularly in what's called the face area – the fusiform face area. The reason it's called the face area is because most people in the population have a visual expertise when it comes to recognising faces. In this case we were finding that it was a little more adapted to baseball pitches in the case of baseball players.'

As well as finding that the brain 'lit up' in the visual and motor cortex areas when the players guessed pitches correctly, Sherwin and Muraskin found that for incorrect guesses the neural activity moved to the prefrontal cortex, which is used for higher-level decision-making and more conscious thought. This suggests that when the automatic, 'System 1' thinking fails, other experience and higher-level thinking gets brought in to figure out why.

'Knowing the neural circuits involved in the rapid decision-making that occurs in baseball opens up the possibility for players to train themselves using their own neural signatures,' said Paul Sajda, who helped co-ordinate the early research at Columbia.

Players can use the data to target their training towards the pitches that are giving them the most trouble. 'Think of it like a diabetic who takes a blood glucose measurement,' says Sherwin. 'You've got to measure your blood glucose level in order to know what your diet is going to be for the rest of the day.'

Although Sherwin is keen to stress that this technology is in its infancy, according to his data targeted training seems to work. On a second visit to one of the college teams they're working with, deCervo found that the decision marker in the brain – the telltale pattern of EEG activity when players recognise a pitch – had moved a little bit further forward in time. The players they had previously tested were using their attention more precisely, homing in on the relevant differences between a fastball and a slider sooner, and this was showing up in their brain activity.

There's even more tantalising potential for deCervo's research. In addition to the computer program they've implemented to measure brain activity using EEG, Sherwin and Muraskin are developing smartphone and tablet apps to help track how people's neural profiles change over time. Sherwin suggests that teams could use it before or during games to see which of their hitters is seeing the ball particularly well that day. The app will also give young players the ability to compare their reaction times to the average major league player, and to use computer-based pitch-recognition tasks to focus their training on the specific areas they need to improve to match them.

Another aim is to build a database of neural profiles which could be used for scouting purposes. There are a number of promising hitters at high school or college level who struggle to make the step up to the major leagues. They might have the bat speed and the strength, but if they can't read and recognise pitches with that extra bit of zip on them, they've got no chance.

This technology could help identify those who can, and prevent careers like that of Billy Beane, who had a batting average of .501 in his first two years of college and was drafted in the first round by the New York Mets. He failed to adapt to the major leagues, however, averaging just .201. Beane would become famous as general manager of the Oakland As and the face of the statistical revolution in baseball detailed in Michael Lewis' book *Moneyball.*

Neuroscience could be the next revolution, but the old guard are as doubtful now as they were then. Sherwin relays a conversation he had with a sceptical scout on a visit to a college in Illinois. 'He said something in the end which really sums up the whole *Moneyball* thing, which was: "I know a good hitter when I see one."

'And I said, "Yeah, but you and 20 other scouts know a good hitter when you see one. How are you really going to do scouting, really find untapped talent if everybody else is there too?"

'There could be a kid who has never played baseball in his life who is amazing at picking up sliders. He could be living in another part of the world where baseball diamonds don't even exist, where they only exist on TV. Instead of looking for the million-dollar arm, we could be looking for the million-dollar brain.'

Your Codename Is: Helix

Upstairs from the Footbonaut at Hoffenheim's training ground, there's a small room with a unique screen inside. It curves around in a semi-circle, with six projectors creating the image of a virtual football pitch. It's called the HELIX, Mayer tells me with a wry smile – an idea from the club's sponsors SAP – and to be fair, if you've got something this cool, you've got to give it a decent codename.

The HELIX is designed to train 'strategic multiple-object tracking', and it's another one of the tools Hoffenheim have been employing to try to give their players an edge. There's crowd noise being piped in through speakers in the darkened space. It's only later, as I watch my beloved AFC Bournemouth labouring to an incredibly dull 0-0 draw in a pre-season friendly at Hoffenheim's Rhein-Neckar Arena, that I realise it was authentic chants from Hoffenheim's own fans. But that's the only hint of realism in what is quite a graphically basic simulation of football. Still, at the moment it's unique: this is the only system of its kind in the world set up specifically for training football players.

Mayer instructs me to stand in the centre of the room, a vantage point from which the screen is so wide that I can't see it all without turning my head. This is crucial. He taps away on another iPad, and four stick-figure players appear on screen – just the outline of a head, torso and two legs straight together. It feels like I've been shrunk down and dropped into a game of table football.

Two of the players are highlighted with flashing red outlines at the start of the game, and my job is to track them as they move around the screen at different angles and speeds. At the end, they all stop, their shirt numbers flash up, and I have to tell Mayer which two players were the ones picked out at the start by telling him the shirt numbers. It gets harder – there are more players to track, a ball to keep an eye on, and even the movement of a referee to distract you. Towards the end it becomes impossible to keep all the players straight in my head and I'm essentially just shouting out four random numbers.

Like Daniel Kahneman, Mayer makes the distinction between fast 'automatic' thinking and slow conscious thinking. 'I think fast thinking is playing the ball, getting a good tackle in, one-on-one tricks, all that stuff,' he says. 'But it is not possible to make everything that is necessary in soccer automatic. I don't think it should be the aim to get tactical decisions automatic – they should be flexible. That is slow thinking.'

Mayer's goals at Hoffenheim are to optimise subconscious fast thinking, which is what the Footbonaut is supposed to do, and to make slow thinking as fast as possible, which is where devices like the HELIX can help. He grins. '*Fast* slow thinking.'

The HELIX trains multiple-object tracking, which is one facet of executive function – a wide umbrella of mental abilities that covers working memory, planning and reasoning, flexibility and problem-solving. Executive function has been linked to success in many areas of life, including sport. One study with youth players from a top division Dutch football club found that their scores on tests of executive function could separate them from amateur players nine times out of 10.

Arthur Kramer, a psychology professor at the University of Illinois, went to Brazil's Centre for the Development of Volleyball, where he and colleagues tested 87 of their best players on their executive function. It includes the ability to hold two different sets of instructions in your head and switch between them; for example, switching between being on the defensive side and the attacking side in a volleyball match as the ball goes back and forth over the net. It also covers being able to stop a task when new information comes up; for example, having to change a tactic quickly based on the actions of the other team. 'We found that athletes were generally able to inhibit behaviour, to stop quickly when they had to, which is very important in sport and in daily life,' said Kramer. 'They were also able to activate, to pick up information from a glance and to switch between tasks more quickly than non-athletes.'

Tests of executive function have also been used to select athletes. When Valeriy Lobanovskyi announced the Soviet Union's football squad for the 1988 European Championships, the press reaction was one of confusion. Lobanovskyi had used computerised testing to select 20 of the players, and his computer had chosen some odd names. This was something the renowned coach had pioneered during his successful spells at Dynamo Kiev, one of the powerhouses of European football at the time. Despite the scepticism, the Soviet Union reached the final of Euro 88, falling only to the brilliance of the Netherlands and Marco van Basten.

In *Football Against the Enemy*, Simon Kuper got first-hand experience of some of the tests, as they were in the early 1990s. There were tests of timing, in which the players had to press a key just as a moving dot crossed a particular line on the screen. There were tests of endurance, in which players had to press one key as many times as they could in 40 seconds, and tests of memory, in which the screen was divided into nine squares with a different number appearing in each. The players had to memorise the numbers and type them in, which was intended to test their ability to remember the positions of players on the pitch.

'The last test I found impossible,' writes Kuper. 'A dot would trace a complicated trajectory through a maze, and then I had to retrace the path, using a joystick. But I could never remember the route, and the maze was so narrow and mazy, and moreover constantly in motion, that I was always bumping into walls. It was, of course, a test of coordination and memory, and it made me realise how extraordinary professional footballers are. Not after years of practice could I have negotiated that maze.'

That last line may not be strictly true. Executive function can be trained. Outside the HELIX room, there's an odd-looking grey workstation – not unlike what I had imagined the computer Kuper did his Soviet tests on to look like. It's called the DT-Wiener Testsystem, and it has been a favourite of cognitive psychologists for decades. In Germany, you have to take a test on it if you lose your driving licence, so some of the players recognise it, says Mayer. I think he's joking.

Most of the team hate it. 'It's the hardest four minutes in the whole year,' Mayer explains. Four minutes later, I can see why.

The system itself is fairly straightforward. It consists of a standard grey computer monitor – the kind you might have had in your office until about 2003. To either side of that is an array of small LEDs which test your peripheral vision. There are two foot switches underneath like the pedals of a car, and, instead of a keyboard, there's a console with an array of coloured buttons and a couple of grey ones – a 1980s arcade machine meets a Fisher-Price children's toy.

There are a variety of stimuli to react to as quickly as possible. I have to press coloured buttons in response to circles flashing up on the screen, push one of the pedals when a particular symbol comes up, or react to high or low tones by pushing one of the grey bars to silence them. It seems to last forever.

I manage to get 295 correct decisions in my four-minute slot. The best players, Mayer tells me, manage to get around 350 correct decisions during their four minutes, with a reaction time of between 0.5 and 0.8 seconds, which Mayer reckons still comes under the 'slow-thinking umbrella' because it's not automatic or subconscious.

Crucially, the players show an improvement over time, despite rarely training on the machine itself. 'We play very fast-paced soccer at Hoffenheim,' says Mayer. 'Even when they don't train with our tool at all they develop from year to year with this fast slow thinking. We think our training philosophy teaches you this while training on the field.'

NeuroTracker is a computer program that poses a very similar challenge to Hoffenheim's HELIX, albeit less sport specific. Since 2012, it has been incorporated into the NFL Scouting Combine, which assesses players on a number of physical and mental criteria before the draft. NeuroTracker measures and trains the brain's ability to track multiple objects – useful if you're a quarterback trying to simultaneously follow the movements of your receivers and any opposition players coming towards you.

Athletes start off sitting in front of a screen, on which a number of balls are displayed against a blank background, moving in different directions – it looks a bit like an old Windows screensaver. Four of the balls are 'target balls' and the athlete's task is to keep track of where they move to and then identify them at the end of the sequence. They do this 20 times over the course of three to five minutes, and that's a complete training session.

As they progress, athletes can make it harder for themselves by introducing physical elements alongside the training, such as standing up instead of sitting down, balancing on something, or, to use an example initiated by an ice hockey team, by skating on a treadmill while controlling a puck. Doing these things while completing the task helps train the brain to track multiple objects without using up too much mental bandwidth.

The key, says the program's developer Jocelyn Faubert, is training the brain's attention system, which is one facet of executive function. 'Players feel that they can see things differently,' he said. 'That is the best feedback possible and why the technology has spread so quickly.'

The system is currently being used by teams in the Premier League, the NFL, the Top 14 of French rugby, and across varsity teams at American universities. It has also been used by Olympic shooting gold medallists, and former taekwondo world number one Aaron Cook, who recorded some of the highest scores ever seen on the software.

NeuroTracker training has a number of advantages, according to Faubert. It helps improve and widen a player's visual field, giving them more information to work with when making decisions. It also makes movement tracking more efficient, freeing up the brain to focus on other tasks, while still keeping an eye on where teammates and opponents are. For example, a footballer could focus his attention on a single opponent's movements to try to anticipate the flight of a shot, without losing track of where other players are in case of a pass.

In a study published in the journal *Nature*, Faubert and his colleagues used NeuroTracker to test and train 102 professional athletes over a number of sessions, including 51 Premier League players, 21 NHL players and 30 rugby players from the French Top 14. They compared them to amateurs and university level sportsmen, and found that the professionals were able to start the program at much higher speeds and improved more quickly than the other groups.

NeuroTracker ability seems to be linked to success in sport as well. A recent study of basketball players found a correlation between scores on multiple-object tracking software and the number of assists and steals during a game in the NBA. Faubert has also tested improvements on the pitch with Premier League players. 'We separated the soccer players into groups,' he said. 'We did the NeuroTracker training and measured their ability to do passing and decision-making on the pitch and they [the group who did the training] improved while the other groups did not improve.'

Athletes can improve their anticipation, decision-making and executive function by training on a computer. Other technology, such as the Footbonaut or the software developed by Axon Sports, is making training more efficient by increasing athletes' exposure to stimuli. This needn't be confined to the elite level; the principles that govern tools such as the Footbonaut can easily be applied to your own sporting endeavours: find out what athletes do differently, and find a way to train it more efficiently.

If it's in The Game, it's in The Game

Mark Cavendish is a tough sprint cyclist, fiercely competitive and outspoken, so it's slightly incongruous to think of him kicking back with a puzzle after a hard day in the saddle. But he too is aware of the importance of keeping his mental skills sharp and, according to an interview in the *Financial Times*, he does it with puzzles such as Sudoku, Slitherlink and Hanidoku. 'Every rider trains their muscles but few train their brain,' he said. 'In a sprint you make 100 decisions a second. What if X goes now and Y goes then? Should I take this gap or that one? You have to be sharp. Over time it becomes instinct. Some riders start screaming. I'm cold, clinical. I swear my heartbeat is 20 or 30 beats slower than theirs.'

Cavendish's love of puzzle games proves that you don't need expensive VR goggles to train your brain. In the next chapter, we'll look at how clever coaches are using our new knowledge of how the brain works to unlock its hidden power. But these advantages aren't just for elite athletes. Brain-training technology is trickling down to the amateur sportsperson as well. If you have a computer or an iPad, you can already try out many of the tools I've mentioned.

Axon Sports, for example, offer a tablet version of their American football training software. Budding quarterbacks can download it, buy the drills for the area they wish to focus on for as little as $5, and train their brain from the comfort of their sofa. It is early days, but as Axon Sports and their partners in the UK develop more training tools for a wider variety of sports, there's no reason why they can't continue to release simplified versions of their software to amateur athletes for football, cricket or tennis.

You may not even need to go that far. Just playing normal video games could train your brain for sport. One study asked 10 college students with little video gaming experience to play war simulation game *Medal of Honor* for 10 days in a row. They found improvements in memory and attention, even on tasks the students hadn't practised.

It turns out that switching attention between various facets of the game – tracking mission objectives, incoming enemies and remaining ammunition – was a perfect way to train control of attention in a wider way.

IntelliGym started life as a game called *Space Fortress*, which was used by the Israeli air force to train fighter pilots. It simulates high-speed decision-making, with the goal of making decisions instinctive. The basic program has been adapted for basketball and hockey – for $12 a month, you can download it to your computer.

The basketball version resembles an early arcade game like *Asteroids*, albeit with a few more bells and whistles. Coloured spaceships move around the screen. Some form part of the player's fleet, while others are enemies, and the player has to safely negotiate the danger using the keyboard. The game activates the same areas of the brain that are involved in decision-making in a real sporting context, and is recommended for use three times a week in 30-minute sessions. The difficulty and nature of the tasks are tailored to the player's strengths and weaknesses, and change over time as the player improves at the game. The hockey version of the program is in use by over 10,000 youth players, as well as professionals in the NHL. Its makers claim that IntelliGym leads to a 30 per cent increase in goals, assists and completed passes within one season.

Of course, digital simulations of sport have been around for decades, although they are designed first and foremost for entertainment value. It is tempting to think that simply sinking hours into the *FIFA* series could yield improvements in performance on the football pitch. *FIFA* players themselves seem to think the game has a knock-on effect: a survey of over 10,000 players at the FIFA Interactive World Cup found that 58 per cent of them felt their on-field performances had been improved by playing *FIFA 12* on the PlayStation 3. There's more: 46 per cent thought the game had improved their understanding of real-life football tactics; 23 per cent credit the game with improving their ball skills; and 17 per cent thought it gave them better awareness of other players on the pitch. They may be on to something. But could cognitive training tools or computer simulations actually replace the dedicated practice that's normally required to reach an elite level in sport?

Jann Mardenborough's life had reached a bit of a dead end. It was the winter of 2009, and the 19-year-old had just dropped out of university and was living with his parents in Wales, making a bit of money selling used car parts on eBay. If he had one passion in life, it was the racing game *Gran Turismo*. From the age of eight onwards, he had put at least two hours a day into the game after school and at friends' houses. For his sixth-form technology project, he had built himself a racing rig for the game out of MDF wood, a gaming wheel and pedals he bought with some Christmas money, and a £20 second-hand Alfa Romeo seat he bought from a scrapyard.

Mardenborough didn't have much in the way of real racing experience – a few visits to an indoor karting track for birthday parties was about the extent of it. But one morning in early 2010, he fired up his PlayStation to find a banner for a competition within *Gran Turismo 5* – compete online against others and win a shot in a real racing car.

More than 90,000 players entered from across Europe, but Mardenborough won.

'It felt completely normal,' says Mardenborough of his first experience of a real racing car at Silverstone, part of his prize. 'I was controlling it just with the throttle and it was completely natural to me.

'The first time I drove anything powerful was during the national finals of GT Academy at Brands Hatch,' he tells me. 'Before the finals I was on eBay looking for some racing boots. I wanted to make a good impression, so I bought these boots on eBay for about £16 all in. I drove a Nissan 370 – we had three goes and we were timed across the final run.

'Drifting this car, 300 horsepower felt amazing. There was a long right-hand corner near the end and on the last run I kept it pinned, and had the car sideways. I'd never been sideways before in my life up until this point, and all I was doing was controlling the slide how I would back home on my steering wheel. It was so exciting, there was so much adrenaline running through me. I was like, "I want to do that as a job."'

He got some formal training, and was given time to adapt to things. 'The feeling you have from your backside as the car is going sideways is completely alien,' he says. 'That took quite a few weeks to fully adapt to.'

In certain areas, he had some catching up to do on drivers who got their hours in more traditional ways. 'I didn't feel it at the time, but you don't have the experience, you don't have the knowledge. Racing in the wet is a completely different feeling you have – there's a lot more variables,' he says. 'We're always at a disadvantage because you just don't have the seat time compared to karters. But what we do have is a lot of race craft – we spent all of our time back home racing against people live across the world.'

Three years later, after some promising performances in smaller racing series, Mardenborough was drinking very real champagne on a very real podium at Hockenheim, having won in GP3 for the first time. In 2015 he made his first tentative step up to GP2, with the aim of eventually driving a Formula 1 car. He has raced at some of the world's most famous circuits, places he already knew well because of hours spent in their virtual equivalents. He had his dream job, and it all started with *Gran Turismo*, training and changing his brain in exactly the same way as racing a real car would have. 'I'd never even power-steered a car before,' he said. 'I had only ever done it in a game.' Mardenborough had made it as a professional sportsperson, without 10,000 hours of real-world practice.

Try this at home:

TRAINING SMARTER

Make your training more efficient

You don't have to have expensive technology like the Footbonaut – just find a way to maximise the number of times you get to perform your skill, whether it's bowling a cricket ball or controlling a football. Smaller-sided games on smaller pitches give each player greater opportunity to interact with the ball, for example.

Train without the meter running

Find out what experts do differently. Home in on it, and try to find a way of exposing yourself to that stimulus but more efficiently. Depending on your sport, there is a variety of software that can help. Axon Sports have apps available to download for American football and baseball, and are developing new software for football and rugby too.

Target transferable skills

There are also training tools that claim to improve your sporting performance more generally. There is some evidence that training executive functions such as multiple-object tracking can improve performance on the field. The NeuroTracker software is probably out of reach of individuals, but programs such as IntelliGym can be downloaded for relatively little.

Cyclist Mark Cavendish swears by Sudoku. The jury is still out, but if you're going to be playing computer games anyway, why not try one that could make you better at sport? It worked for gamer-turned-racer Jann Mardenborough.

CHAPTER FIVE

UNLOCKING THE BRAIN'S HIDDEN POWER

Gary Neville is, if it's possible, even more of a prickly character in retirement than he was during his years as a combative right-back for Manchester United. He has been dabbling in the leisure industry, and I meet him at Hotel Football, a venture he co-owns with Ryan Giggs and other members of United's famous Class of 92. From the five-a-side pitch on the roof, you get a unique view over Old Trafford, the club's famous stadium – it's fitting when you consider the plaudits Neville has won for his own fresh perspective on football during his punditry work for Sky Sports. Between giving me his views on the media, video technology and the state of Premier League defending for a piece in *Sport* magazine, Neville tells me something interesting about the rehabilitation process at Manchester United. 'We used to have an eye specialist, going back 15 years,' he says. 'At the time I didn't listen to her, but now I think she's right. When you're not match fit, what that can mean is two things. One is physically you can be a little bit down, but the other is the idea of being able to use your eyes to be sharp.'

Peripheral-vision training is used to help players retain their mental match sharpness. It's just one of the ways in which athletes are adopting new technologies to unlock the power of their brains that we'll take a look at in this chapter.

'We used to have machines, and I'm sure they still have them at Carrington, where we used to do eye-training sessions,' says Neville. 'When you come back from being injured and when you're out for a long time, "match fit" isn't just your legs and your ability to run; it's other elements like the sharpness, the repetitive elements in your head. Your instinct has gone a little bit because your eyes are untrained.'

The eye specialist Neville is referring to is Professor Gail Stephenson, who sadly passed away in July 2015. She was a favoured aide to Sir Alex Ferguson through much of his reign at United – reportedly, it was her feedback that caused him to change his side out of an infamous grey away kit and into blue and white at half-time during a 3-1 defeat to Southampton in April 1996. 'In soccer, improving the way players use their eyes can improve both the quality of the information their eyes receive and the speed they process the information,' she said in an interview with the *Manchester Evening News* in 2010. 'Therefore the quicker they instigate the action, the more effective they will be during a game. Approximately 80 per cent of the information we use to make any decision for an action comes from vision. The average person uses their eyes to only about 50 per cent of their full potential, so exercising certain aspects of that vision can increase the percentage and, in some instances, improve an individual's quality of life.'

Vision can be trained. The software can, in some cases, improve the hardware. In this chapter, we'll look at how training with new technology can unlock hidden aspects of not just vision, but every facet of an athlete's brain.

Some of the tools we've already seen can help train peripheral vision. Hoffenheim's HELIX screen has boosted some of their players' visual field from 180 degrees to 200 degrees. Visual acuity can also be improved, according to Aaron Seitz and Daniel Ozer at the University of California, Riverside. They have developed a tool called UltimEyes, which is available for download as a tablet and smartphone app for only a few pounds. It doesn't look like much – just a grey background with some faint grey blobs called Gabor patches on it. It reminded me of blurry images from biology textbooks showing plant cells under a microscope.

You sit a metre and a half (nearly five feet) away from the screen. There are different types of task: in some you see four shapes in different orientations, and you have to click on the one that matches a target shape. In another, you simply have to click on all the shapes that you can see as quickly as possible. What is common across all the tasks is that they get harder as you go through – the shapes get fainter, or the lines on them decrease in thickness. The creators recommend four sessions a week, and claim that doing this training for two months could allow you to see two lines further down on one of the letter charts used in eye tests.

'We're using the brain as glasses,' says Uri Polat, the creator of an iPhone app that also uses Gabor patches to train vision, although GlassesOff is targeted at older people who want to delay the need for reading glasses. The improvement is nothing to do with strengthening eye muscles, or enhancing the retina, it's all about training the brain – improving the ability of the visual processing areas of the brain (feature detector neurons) to detect lines and edges.

Before the 2013 college baseball season, Seitz and Ozer split the Highlanders, UC Riverside's team, into two groups. One group received 30 x 25-minute visual training sessions on what would eventually become the UltimEyes software, while the other group received no training. The visual acuity of the test group improved by 31 per cent – some of them saw their vision improve to 20/7.5 (with 20/20 being normal uncorrected vision) – and they felt their vision had improved while reading, driving or watching TV as well.

The results on the pitch were equally remarkable. The test group saw their strikeouts fall by 4.4 per cent, while their improvement in batting average, slugging percentage and on-base percentage was three times greater than the average league player over the same period. 'The vision tests demonstrate that training-based benefits transfer outside the context of the computerised training program to standard eye charts,' said Seitz. 'Players reported seeing the ball better, greater peripheral vision and an ability to distinguish lower-contrast objects.'

The Highlanders' coach was impressed too. 'I didn't think we would see as much of an improvement as we did,' said Doug Smith. 'Our guys stopped swinging at some pitches and started hitting at others. Everyone is looking for an edge to be that little bit better. Our guys are more confident now when they come to the plate.'

Perhaps the most telling statistic of all comes from Ozer, who plugged the data into a formula developed by Bill James, the baseball statistician of *Moneyball* fame. He estimated that the visual training task had contributed to four or five extra wins during the course of that season.

A few years ago, Nike developed 'Vapor Strobe' glasses, which work in a similar way to the glasses used by researchers in some of the occlusion studies of anticipation that we looked at in the first part of the book. The glasses rapidly alternate between clear and opaque up to six times per second, which in theory helps train the visual system to see the path of a ball more clearly by forcing it to learn to fill in the gaps.

A study commissioned by Nike and conducted by Duke University in North Carolina tested 500 people across more than 1,200 training sessions using the glasses as they completed tasks such as catching and throwing a ball. 'Our results varied, but stroboscopic training does seem to enhance vision and attention,' said Stephen Mitroff, who worked on the study. 'Not every test we tried showed differences, but several showed significant improvements.' After training with the strobe glasses, the college athletes who took part in the study were more sensitive to small amounts of motion, and better at picking up visual details that were only available for a fraction of a second. This confirms previous research that has found that stroboscopic training, as this technique is called, can improve visual processing, encoding in short-term memory and anticipatory timing (being able to predict when a moving object is going to be at a certain spot) – all important components of athletic performance.

Another study from Duke University compared two groups of professional ice hockey players from the Carolina Hurricanes, an NHL team. During their pre-season training camp in 2011, 11 volunteers from the playing staff were split into two groups. The first group trained normally, while the second group wore the Nike glasses for at least 10 minutes a day for 16 days, while they carried out their normal training camp activities, both on and off the ice. Before they started training, both groups undertook a test designed by their coaches. Forwards had to collect a puck placed on an X two feet from the goal line, skate a figure of eight with the puck, and then take a shot at the empty goal. They were awarded one point for each successful shot, for a possible total of 20 points. Defenders had a similar task that involved a long pass towards the red line at the opposite end of the ice.

After 16 days of training, all the players took the test again. Every player who had been wearing the strobe glasses improved their score, with an 18 per cent increase on average, while only two members of the control group got better. Tantalising though these findings are, it's not quite time to start equipping every athlete in the country with a pair of strobe glasses. For a start, Nike no longer make them. 'There are still many open questions,' said Mitroff. 'We don't know how long these effects last. We don't know how much training is needed, and we don't yet have the whole picture on what is being trained.'

That hasn't stopped professional teams from trying it out, though. In an interview with *TED*, former NFL punter Chris Kluwe explained their benefits when used in practice. 'It is mainly for the receivers training to focus on the balls coming in and predict where the ball was going to be, even if they couldn't watch it the entire way in,' he said. 'When you're running on the field, when you're trying to fight the defensive back, then you're not going to be able to just stare the ball all the way into your hands. You have to predict where it's going to end up, and then know when to close your hands to catch it.'

Look Where The Best Look

Dr Joan Vickers is perhaps the world's leading expert on where athletes look to collect advance information. The Canadian scientist has fitted athletes across a wide range of sports with eye trackers, and she's found that the best athletes in the world all tend to use their eyes in similar ways – ways that are distinct and different from non-experts. In one experiment, she asked two groups of gymnasts to look at a series of slides from a video of someone performing on a balance beam. The highly skilled gymnasts made fewer eye movements, but made them for longer, and tended to focus on the athlete's torso, whereas the lower skilled athletes looked at the gymnast's head, feet and hands. One study of basketball free-throw shooters found that experts looked at the hoop for almost a second on their successful attempts, while non-experts fixated on the target for just 400 milliseconds. Across a broad range of sports, from shooting to tennis to baseball to football, elite athletes make fewer eye movements and look at the target for longer before they initiate an action.

Vickers has dubbed this phenomenon the 'quiet eye', and in her own words it's something she's been 'obsessed' with since her days as a talented college athlete. 'I was fortunate in university to play in not one but two varsity teams – basketball and volleyball – the whole four years I was there,' she says. 'I remember consciously becoming aware that how I controlled my visual attention was critical in those sports. I remember the moment when I realised that if you don't control this precise information that you have to have at this precise moment then that skill is not going to work very well.'

Just like Cristiano Ronaldo in chapter one, the best athletes across a range of sports can be differentiated from amateurs by the way they use the quiet eye to quickly collect the advance visual cues they need to react accurately. 'The place that elite athletes look in reading a pitch, reading a serve, reading the puck coming off the stick, it's always the same,' Vickers tells me over the phone from her office at the University of Calgary. 'It's in front of the object. Imagine you're looking across a tennis court and you want to see the serve coming off the racket. You're going to put your gaze slightly in front, so you're able to see the ball, but also see the complete swing and movement of the person as they are making the delivery.'

This seems obvious, but it's something that some amateur athletes are really bad at. 'I tested a girl in golf who had a terrible time putting,' says Vickers. 'She'd bought five of the best putters in the world. We put the eye tracker on her and at first we thought it was broken actually, because for 22 minutes she never fixated the ball once, and never fixated the hole. It's hard to believe, but she had no awareness that how she controlled her visual attention and her focus actually had anything to do with her ability to putt.'

The quiet eye is not a fixed or innate ability, it can be trained; and, of all the techniques in the book, it is the one that perhaps has the potential to create the most striking impact and improvement for amateur athletes in a short space of time. Leighann Doan is testament to that. While she was at college, the basketball player's free throws were wildly inconsistent. She would be at 100 per cent in some games, but in others her success rate was down nearer 40 per cent. Luckily, her college was the University of Calgary, so she became one of the first athletes to benefit from Vickers' expertise.

There are a number of steps to developing a quiet-eye training programme for a new sport or skill, Vickers tells me. First, get eye trackers on the best athletes in the world. This is getting much easier as technology improves. There's a PBS documentary from around 10 years ago with actor Alan Alda looking at Vickers' work. In it, she's using eye trackers on ice hockey players, what with it being Canada and all. They equip the players with big helmets, heavier than the ones they normally wear, with wires trailing from the back of them to a computer at the side of the ice. Each tracked player has to have two cable wranglers skating along behind them, holding the wire so that it doesn't get tangled up in their skates. It looks like a recipe for disaster.

Times have changed. Last year, four engineering students at Georgia Tech college in the US managed to incorporate an eye-tracking device into a quarterback's helmet. Using some smart software, they can project a cone on to footage, showing a quarterback's visual field based on their head and eye movements.

Vickers' next step is to develop a prototype showing exactly where the experts look when they execute their skills. Then, you bring in the people you want to train and show them videos of where the best players in the world look.

To encourage them to keep their gaze fixated on the right target, coaches can ask the athletes they're training to say a set phrase out loud before taking a shot – something like 'Sight, focus' has been used for basketball. The words themselves don't matter; it's just that saying them makes sure the player's gaze is actually on the target for at least a second. Everything seems to fall into place from there. The body naturally aligns its movements with the gaze; people stop focusing too much on body mechanics and let their natural instincts take over. Try it next time you play basketball, mini golf or even pool.

In Leighann Doan's case, the improvement was remarkable. 'Instead of just looking at the hoop, I had now learned to select a very specific spot on the rim and focus my eyes there for only a very short time,' she wrote in an article for PBS. 'It was not important what spot I chose as long as I was able to focus on it every time. Different shooters choose different locations as their targets, some the back of the rim, others the front of the rim and still others choose the middle of the rim. For me, I chose the back of the rim, more specifically the notch where the mesh is tied to the rim. This gave me a spot I could immediately locate on every hoop and thus perfect my routine. The importance of the routine is to have the same shot every time. How can one expect to have a high free-throw percentage when one never knows what the shot will look like? By having a specific routine, doing the same action every shot and focusing on the same spot every time, I had a much higher chance of my shot being the same every time.'

Her free-throw accuracy increased to 80 per cent, and she went on to play for Canada's national team and carve out a professional career in Europe. 'The theory of quiet eye has helped me to become a better all-around player,' she writes. 'There is always room for improvement in my game and it is often the little things that make the biggest difference. Becoming a better free-throw shooter adds another dimension to my game and allows me to face the high-pressure challenge on the free-throw line with greater confidence. Before learning of this technique, it was always a guessing game as to why my free-throw shooting was only average. Now I have a very simple yet profound skill that allows me to monitor my shot.'

The Original Brain-Training Tool

Mike Cammalleri looks like a man possessed. His eyes dart from side to side, and the hockey stick in his hand turns with them, waiting for the right moment to strike. It's the Eastern Conference semi-finals of ice hockey's Stanley Cup in 2010, and things are delicately poised between the Pittsburgh Penguins and Cammalleri's Montreal Canadiens. The seven-game series is tied 3-3, so this will be the decider.

Cammalleri is a short but strong left wing with closely cropped dark hair. He leads the scoring charts in the play-offs so far, but with this tricky decider in unfriendly territory, the Canadiens need him more than ever if they're going to reach their first conference final for 18 years. He picks his spot, picks his moment and, with a final, powerful flick of the wrist, he dispatches the puck goalwards.

Except the game hasn't started yet. Hours before this deciding match-up, this is what television cameras caught Cammalleri doing on the bench. An old-school brain-training tool. He was looking at a spot out on the rink, visualising what he was going to do if he got the puck in that position. It worked. At the start of the second period, he picked up possession near the halfway line, drove forward, eyes darting left and right, and with a flick of the wrist dispatched the puck into the net.

We rarely get to see visualisation in such vivid detail; normally, it happens in the privacy of an athlete's home, or in the dressing room before a game. But it has become increasingly prevalent, almost ubiquitous in elite level sport. 'Part of my preparation is I go and ask the kit man what colour we're wearing – if it's red top, white shorts, white socks or black socks,' said Wayne Rooney. 'Then I lie in bed the night before the game and visualise myself scoring goals or doing well. You're trying to put yourself in that moment and trying to prepare yourself, to have a "memory" before the game. I don't know if you'd call it visualising or dreaming, but I've always done it, my whole life. When I was younger, I used to visualise myself scoring wonder goals, stuff like that. From 30 yards out, dribbling through teams. You used to visualise yourself doing all that, and when you're playing professionally, you realise it's important for your preparation.'

Jessica Ennis-Hill used visualisation to help her win gold in the heptathlon at the 2012 Olympics. 'I use visualisation to think about the perfect technique,' she said. 'If I can get that perfect image in my head, then hopefully it'll affect my physical performance.' Rugby player Jonny Wilkinson used it before crucial penalty kicks for England. 'I visualise the ball travelling along that path and imagine the sensation of how the ball is going to feel when it hits my foot for the perfect strike,' he has said.

People have probably always used it to prepare for big events, but visualisation, or imagery as it's often called, was first formalised by the Soviet Union's Olympic coaches, and is thought to have played an important part in their successes in the mid-20th century (alongside some other clandestine techniques, perhaps). In his book *Peak Performance*, Dr Charles Garfield cites a study conducted by Soviet sports psychologists in the lead-up to the 1980 Winter Olympics at Lake Placid, where the USSR won twice as many medals as the USA.

Athletes were split into four groups, who practised for the same amount of time, but with varying ratios of visualisation to physical practice. Those in the group that had done the least amount of physical practice and the most visualisation were the ones who showed the greatest improvement. Other studies with basketball and darts players have found that a group who simply visualised improved as much as a group who actually practised for the same amount of time.

Imagery has become ever more sophisticated since then. 'Back in the 1980s, in the Wild West days, it really was just a case of getting the athlete to sit down and close their eyes and visualise themselves performing,' says Dr Steve Bull, who worked with the England cricket team and has now taken his visualisation techniques to the business world. When he was first introducing the idea to dressing rooms, there was some resistance to what was then seen as a rather fanciful notion. But Bull would watch cricketers shadowing shots in the dressing room or between deliveries – a form of visualisation – and realised that the techniques were already being used by athletes, just in informal ways.

It's important, when visualising, for the mental imagery to be as vivid as possible, to incorporate as many senses as possible – sounds, smell and touch as well as sight. It's why Rooney asks the kit man what shirts United will be wearing that weekend. 'Desmond Haynes, the famous West Indian batter, used to tell a very powerful story about the fact that he'd never scored a hundred at the WACA in Perth,' Bull tells me. 'The day before a Test match he walked out into the middle and he looked around the ground, no one in it of course, and he visualised himself scoring the hundred. He raised his bat and then he walked back to the pavilion to this imaginary applause, and lo and behold he went out there the next day and scored his first career hundred at Perth.'

Visualisation works because it recruits the same neural circuits that the brain uses for action. Thinking about a particular action makes completing that action in future more likely because, remember, neurons that fire together wire together. One study measured muscle impulses in skiers as they used visualisation and found the same pattern of electrical activity you would expect if they were actually performing. This extends incredibly far: Alvaro Pascual-Leone found that pianists simply thinking about playing a sequence of keys had long-term changes to their cortical maps.

Visualisation can even change the body. One remarkable study found that simply thinking about lifting weights actually increased muscle strength. In that experiment, the group doing physical training increased their strength by 53 per cent, but those who merely imagined doing it still saw a 35 per cent increase in strength. Admittedly, this was only in finger strength, but in a similar experiment involving visualising bicep curls participants showed a 13.5 per cent improvement without ever picking up a weight.

The latest research shows that it is probably a good idea to move around a little bit, even if you are just visualising. A study of elite high jumpers by Professor Aymeric Guillot at the University of Lyon found that mental imagery improved jump success and form by 35 per cent, while those rehearsing the jump as much as they could without actually jumping improved by 45 per cent. Dry runs are useful, whether it's taking a practice swing at the tee or playing fake shots on your way to the crease – it all gets the brain ready for action.

New technology is making it even easier for athletes to create vivid, accurate imagery. Video screens are everywhere and, with systems like Prozone, it's simpler than ever for athletes to get detailed footage of their own performances. Efforts are also ongoing to make other brain-training tools more realistic and complex, and this will only continue as creating a virtual reality environment becomes more accessible with devices such as Oculus Rift. Dr Cathy Craig at Queen's University Belfast has worked with Ulster Rugby club to create an immersive, interactive virtual environment where players' perceptual skills can be tested in a similar way to some of the touch-screen-based tools we've looked at. The player wears a backpack full of sensors and a head-mounted display. 'The advantages of this technology are that, unlike playing a video game on a normal desktop computer, the rugby player or athlete is totally immersed in a realistic simulated environment,' she said. 'By presenting stereoscopic images in a head-mounted display and tracking head movements, the user's viewpoint is automatically updated, giving a 360-degree virtual experience. This means that the user becomes totally absorbed in their virtual environment, encouraging them to interact as they would in the real world.'

Belgium's Secret

In this chapter and the last, we've looked at a wide range of techniques for training the brain more efficiently and unlocking its power. Research continues, but preliminary findings suggest that training games like the ones developed by NeuroTracker and Axon Sports could complement more established methods such as visualisation and help athletes train their minds without wearing out their bodies. But before these cognitive training tools are widely adopted, they may face the same battle for acceptance as visualisation did 30 years ago.

I should add my own note of caution. There remains scepticism from within the scientific community as to the effectiveness of some of these new tools and techniques. 'There's certainly no magic solution here,' insists Dr Vincent Walsh, one of the world's leading cognitive neuroscientists. 'If you do a brain-training game seven hours a day, all you're going to be becoming better at is a brain-training game. The brain is a modular machine – when you train one bit of it to do something, you are training that one bit of it. The less like the sport it is, the less it transfers.'

Independent research is slowly catching up with the pace of technological development, though, and the early results are promising. In January 2014, Thomas Romeas at the University of Montreal found that multiple-object tracking on computer training software such as Hoffenheim's HELIX or NeuroTracker *can* improve on-field decision-making. A group of players who participated in object-tracking exercises in the lab showed a 15 per cent improvement in their on-field decision-making skills compared to control and placebo groups. That may not sound like much, but when every fraction could mean the difference between winning and losing, it adds up to a lot.

Technology marches on, but some coaches are already ahead of the curve when it comes to incorporating what we know about the brain into their training sessions. When Christian Benteke joined Liverpool in the summer of 2015 for a hefty £32.5m fee, the Belgian striker was feeling the pressure. He had scored plenty of goals in an Aston Villa shirt with his strong and skilful play, but performing in front of the famous Kop end is something else. Expectations were high. The heat was on. So, he picked up the phone and called Michel Bruyninckx.

The Belgian coach has pioneered an approach of 'brain-centred learning' in football – taking what we now know about the brain and using it to design sessions that train it more effectively. While working for Standard Liege, he played an instrumental role in the development of a number of talented Belgian players, including Benteke, Anderlecht midfielder Steven Defour and Napoli striker Dries Mertens. 'He has given me that crucial extra metre in my head that is so important,' Mertens told the BBC.

Bruyninckx's training methods are focused on enhancing plasticity, creating and strengthening connections in the brain and adding myelin to neural pathways to speed up thought. With youth players he uses SenseBall – a small football in a hand-held net which allows players to get many more touches of the ball. 'Normally, a professional player will make about 35,000 touches of the ball per season,' said Bruyninckx in an interview with Belgian TV. 'Now, thanks to SenseBall, if a youngster uses it regularly he or she can reach around 4–500,000 touches per season. It is above all brain speed that will influence actions.'

It's not just about getting more touches of the ball. Bruyninckx's training also aims to overload the brain: players are asked to do several things at once, and rarely do the same session more than two or three times. Bruyninckx has worked closely with former Charlton Athletic and Blackpool boss Jose Riga, and both were called in by AC Milan to help the club develop its home-grown talent. Watching Bruyninckx's drills is striking – the players move in complex patterns, in harmony. Players might be asked to play without boots to enhance their touch in one session, to speak in different languages while doing strength conditioning work, or to do maths puzzles while doing passing drills. In group exercises, overload means that the players are constantly on the move; they have to be concentrating even if they don't have the ball at their feet at that particular moment.

Overloading players during training helps them develop the mental flexibility to cope with the changing demands of their game. It creates adaptable players, like Benteke. 'When he was a boy in Belgium, he changed regularly from one club to another, because he only had one profile – as a physically strong player,' Bruyninckx told the *Mirror*. 'I tried to encourage him then to expand his mind to see that he must not accept those labels and that he could continuously change his skills, and the way he learned to think has been enormously important to his career. I hear people say he is not a Liverpool type of player, but I tell you that he can adapt to any club.'

Kevin McGreskin, who works with Partick Thistle in Scotland, also tries to overload the brain in his Soccer eyeQ training programme. One of his exercises involves asking the youth players he trains to throw a tennis ball and call out colours while they're passing a football. 'Overload exercises help the player speed up the feet and the thought process,' he said in an interview with *The Blizzard*. These techniques are similar to those employed by baseball coach Joe Maddon, who led the Tampa Bay Rays to a division title in 2008 with an unfancied team of young players, as Jonah Keri explains in his book *The Extra 2%*. Instead of the usual pitching machine, Maddon purchased one for smaller tennis balls, reasoning that if hitters could follow a tennis ball at 140mph, then a baseball at 90mph should be no problem. He set the machines to different heights to challenge his hitters' field of vision, and also started marking the balls with red and black ink and asking his players to shout out the colour as the pitch was on its way. It's a technique that keeps athletes pushing at the edges of their ability, sharpens their focus and even trains their visual acuity – the perfect brain-based training tool.

Premier League goalkeeper Petr Cech and his coach Christophe Lollichon have been using this approach at the highest level. 'We try to catch different shape balls, bigger balls or smaller ones because then you need to adapt your hand-eye coordination every time,' said Cech in an interview with the *London Evening Standard*. 'Suddenly your brain starts working again. You can use colours. Imagine you saving the ball but at the same time a card is held up. You save the ball and shout the colour – you are concentrating on more things. That makes your peripheral vision better as well. Your brain is working much more than just with a simple catch.

'He [Lollichon] is always searching for new things to bring it further, to be more efficient and try to make things happen for a goalkeeper to progress even at the highest level. I keep using a table tennis robot which shoots ping-pong balls out. You have to catch it with one hand so it gives you a completely different hand-eye coordination. Then, when you have both hands facing one football, everything becomes easier.'

So far we've seen how methods both old and new are helping athletes improve by making training more efficient, and how you can adopt them to boost your own sporting performances. But, as we'll see in the next two chapters, our growing knowledge of neuroscience can also have an impact at the other end of the scale – when things go wrong.

Try this at home:

UNLOCK YOUR BRAIN'S POTENTIAL

Look in the right place

Your brain knows how to do most things; you just need to give it the right information. The quiet eye potentially has the biggest potential to improve your game overnight. Whether you're playing pool, golf or basketball, simply looking at the target for longer before you start your action can make a huge difference. Try saying out loud a set phrase such as 'Sight, focus' before you take a shot to make sure your eyes stay fixed on the target.

Visualise new pathways

Neurons that fire together wire together, and imagining yourself succeeding at something is a great way to strengthen the neural pathways that will determine that success. Visualisation works better the more realistic it is, so focus on all your senses ahead of big moments, whether in sport or outside it, and concentrate on the details. Feel yourself performing in the way you want to.

Overload your brain

Once you've learnt a skill, you can make it more robust and instinctive by training while performing other tasks at the same time. Coaches have asked their charges to shout out the colour of a dot on the ball as they're catching it. Petr Cech practises catching against a table-tennis robot to sharpen his reflexes and hand-eye co-ordination. Be imaginative – how can you stretch the skills required for your sport?

CHAPTER SIX

LUIS SUAREZ AND THE AMYGDALA HIJACK

It only took a split second. Few watching it live on television will have clocked exactly what had happened off the ball, almost out of shot, in the opening minutes of rugby league's Super League Grand Final at Old Trafford in 2014. But as Ben Flower's conscious brain reseized control, the magnitude of the career-defining mistake he had just made will have slowly dawned on him.

It was a huge occasion between two massive rivals in a sport that's always played with passion and power. As his Wigan side attacked just a minute and a half into the game, Flower was clipped by Lance Hohaia of St Helens – just a glancing blow, but it seemed to trip a switch in Flower's brain and the red mist descended.

After the officials finished separating the players from the ensuing mass brawl, the replays showed the full extent of Flower's brutal attack. The first assault, a swing of a powerful right fist, rendered his opponent unconscious; the second, shocking blow – a punch delivered to the forehead of the prone Hohaia – played out on the big screen to gasps from the 76,000 assembled fans. Flower was sent off and subsequently banned for six months. Hohaia retired from rugby a few months later with recurrent concussion symptoms.

'The first punch was instinct,' said Flower in an interview with the *Guardian* just before he returned to action after his ban. 'I had chased the ball and, potentially, I could have scored. After the frustration of dropping the ball, and getting hit from the side, it's a natural reaction. But with the second punch there was no thought process. It happened so quick you couldn't control it. The hype of the whole week blew up in one overreaction from me. I don't know what I was thinking. It was the perfect sort of place to hit someone.'

It only took a split second, plus a few moments for the marks on the defender's shoulder to fade. A corner, swung in from the left in a World Cup group game between Italy and Uruguay. A tussle, the kind you see dozens of times in your average international game, and then a moment that shocked the world. Uruguay's star striker Luis Suarez, a man with a reputation for crossing the line, had just sunk his teeth into the shoulder of Italian defender Giorgio Chiellini.

It was the third time he had bitten an opponent. The first was while playing for Ajax in 2010, the second victim was Chelsea's Branislav Ivanovic in 2013, and then this incident watched by millions at the 2014 World Cup in Brazil. 'The adrenaline levels in a game can be so high; the pulse is racing and sometimes the brain doesn't keep up,' says Suarez in his 2014 autobiography, *Crossing the Line*. 'The pressure mounts and there is no release valve. In 2010, I was frustrated because we were drawing what was a very important game, and we were on a bad run. I wanted to do everything right that day, and it felt as though I was doing everything wrong. The pent-up frustration and feeling that it was my fault reached a point where I couldn't contain it any more.

'With Ivanovic in 2013, we had to beat Chelsea still to have any chance of making it into the Champions League. I was having a terrible game. I gave away a stupid penalty with a handball and I could feel everything slipping through our fingers. I could feel myself getting wound up. Moments before the Chiellini bite, I had a great chance to put us 1-0 up. If I had scored that goal, if Buffon hadn't made the save, then I would not have done anything. But I missed the chance. When the heart has stopped racing after the game, it's easy to look back and say, "How could you be so stupid? There were 20 minutes left." But out on the pitch with the adrenaline pumping and the tension mounting, you're not even really aware of how long is left. You don't know anything. All I could think was: "I didn't score. We're out of the World Cup." The fear of failure clouds everything for me – even the blatantly obvious fact that I have at least 20,000 pairs of eyes on me; it is not as if I am not going to be seen. Logic doesn't come into it.'

That's literally true – in the case of Suarez, of Flower, of Zinedine Zidane's infamous head butt in the 2006 World Cup final, of Eric Cantona's assault on a fan at Selhurst Park in 1996, of Serena Williams threatening to shove a ball down a line judge's throat. All were caused by an 'amygdala hijack', which is what happens when the brain's instinctive, emotional side seizes control. In this chapter, we'll examine what is happening in the brain when things go wrong, looking at how and why athletes choke, and the dreaded 'yips' – extreme cases of choking which have ended careers.

You have two amygdala, one in each hemisphere of the brain in the temporal lobe, where imaginary lines drawn through your eye and your ear would intersect. They're commonly described as almond-shaped, although if you found an almond that looked like this in your bag of mixed nuts you probably wouldn't risk it. The amygdala plays a key role in decision-making and emotion. It receives input from all the sensory areas of the brain – vision, touch, hearing, taste and smell.

There are two routes to the amygdala. The long route passes through higher cortical areas, so we're consciously aware of what's going on. But there's also a shortcut which bypasses conscious perception. When the amygdala perceives a threat it can send a distress signal directly to the hypothalamus before the brain's higher centres of thought have a chance to process the information for themselves. The hypothalamus triggers the release of adrenaline and other hormones which prepare the body for evasive action by raising the heart rate, sending extra oxygen to the brain and muscles, and sharpening the senses. This results in what is known as the flight, fight or freeze response – an instinctive, hard-wired trigger for dealing with potential danger.

Hail to The Chimp

This response is very helpful when you need to jump out of the way of a speeding car, for example. But, unfortunately, the amygdala can also be hijacked by things that are not genuinely dangerous, such as the pressure of missing a big chance in a crucial World Cup game, or being insulted by an opponent. There are three telltale stages of an amygdala hijack: an emotional reaction, like Luis Suarez getting wound up when he gave away a penalty against Chelsea in 2013; an inappropriate response, like Zinedine Zidane when he head-butted Marco Materazzi; and, later, regret, like Ben Flower in the hours after his assault on Hohaia, when he could be found sobbing in the car park as his conscious mind tried to process the enormity of what he had done.

The amygdala hijack is compounded in certain situations because the operation of the prefrontal cortex is impaired under stress. The prefrontal cortex is involved in many things, including regulating attention and focus and inhibiting inappropriate behaviour, so you can see how it malfunctioning can cause problems on the field. Teenagers and children have less developed prefrontal cortices, which is why they're more prone to behaving like teenagers and children.

Under stress, athletes can revert to that state, resulting in a more emotional reaction and an inability to counteract the amygdala hijack and control the fight, flight or freeze response. We've seen the fight aspect of this above, while freezing might manifest itself as choking under pressure, which we'll discuss at length below. On the field, 'flight' could mean players rushing to get through the stressful situation so it will be over, which can obviously make matters worse. One study of England's penalty shoot-out record found that their players took a lot less time before striking a penalty than the more successful nations. Gareth Southgate admitted as much after his missed penalty put England out of Euro 96. This is a classic symptom of an amygdala hijack.

Trying to interpret the physiological response (heart racing, quick breathing) in a different way could help lessen the consequences of an emotional reaction. In the 1970s, researchers in Canada asked male volunteers to walk across rope bridges, one at 230 feet, above a river in British Columbia. At the end of the bridge, an attractive female accomplice was waiting, who offered the men her phone number in case they wanted to hear more about the project later on.

The higher the bridge, the more likely the men were to give the woman a call. The call-back rate was much less on a lower bridge which didn't evoke the same fear response. The men on the higher bridge had interpreted the physiological stress signals from walking over it as an attraction for the woman. Some even asked her out on a date. It was the bridge, not the woman, that drove the men's responses – but they had unwittingly reinterpreted their physiological symptoms and redirected the course of an amygdala hijack.

Much of the work that traditional sports psychologists do involves teaching athletes to control their emotional side, to reinterpret the signals their body is sending them and try to prevent amygdala hijacks and counteract their effects. Practitioners in this field have gained much greater acceptance across sport in recent years by building models and frameworks based on the brain that are easier for athletes to understand and implement. Dr Steve Peters, a renowned sports psychologist who has worked closely with Liverpool Football Club and snooker star Ronnie O'Sullivan, is one of the best known. His book, *The Chimp Paradox*, is one of the biggest-selling self-help guides of recent years, and in it he suggests that our behaviour is determined by two distinct internal forces: the Human and the Chimp. The Human is the reasoning, rational part of the brain – the prefrontal cortex. The

Chimp is the underlying emotions and behaviours – the amygdala hijacker.

Peters has achieved great success with sportspeople – helping O'Sullivan to battle his inner demons, and former track cyclist Victoria Pendleton to keep her emotions in check – by teaching athletes to control their inner Chimps and find a sense of balance.

New Zealand's fearsome rugby team, the All Blacks, use a different framework with similar goals. The team are formidable; their record is second to none, and they work hard to intimidate their opponents with the haka – an impressive, aggressive pre-match ritual. But despite their excellent record, the All Blacks coaches found that some of their players were finding it difficult to control their emotions during games. With the help of former footballer Ceri Evans, they developed a two-part framework called Red Head/Blue Head to help.

For the players, it involves monitoring their own emotions to identify when they're on the verge of entering 'Red-Head mode', and finding a way of cooling down and getting back into the right mental state. Yes, the haka helps get the All Blacks pumped up for the game, but it also shifts them from Red Head to Blue Head. They use it to reinterpret any nervousness, fear or other physical symptoms they might be feeling because of an amygdala hijack into a more constructive emotion.

Of course, lashing out like Flower or Suarez is just one way that pressure and the amygdala hijack can affect athletes. Most people are relatively good at not physically attacking people when they're under pressure, but nearly all will have seen their performance suffer.

A Nation Chokes

A small step to the right ruined Moacyr Barbosa's life. He was the home goalkeeper in the final game of the 1950 World Cup in Brazil, in front of 200,000 people at the Maracana stadium in Rio de Janeiro – the largest crowd ever assembled for a football match.

Brazil needed only a draw to lift the trophy for the first time in their history, and with just over 10 minutes to go, the game was tied at 1-1. But Uruguayan winger Alcides Ghiggia was racing down the flank. Anticipating a cross like the one that had led to Uruguay's first goal, Barbosa shifted his weight on to his right foot. But instead the ball came in low and hard, inside the near post and past his despairing dive.

He became a scapegoat for the defeat and was vilified as 'the man who made all of Brazil cry'. Despite all the success they've had in World Cups since, the shock loss of the tournament on home soil left a scar on the Brazilian national consciousness. Poet Nelson Rodrigues called it 'our catastrophe, our Hiroshima', but it's better known in Brazil as the '*Maracanazo*' – the Maracana blow.

That was the historical background to the 2014 World Cup, which was meant to be a chance for Brazil to heal those wounds by finally winning the competition on home ground. Instead, in the space of 90 astonishing minutes in the semi-final, it left a fresh wound running just as deep. Once again, Brazil had gone into the competition as strong favourites, but they'd stuttered through the early rounds, and they lost their star player and talisman Neymar to a back injury in the quarter-final against Colombia.

Before the semi-final against Germany, then, the Brazilian anthem rang out with even more passion than usual. Defender David Luiz and goalkeeper Julio Cesar held up a shirt with Neymar's name on it in homage to their injured colleague, as the crowd carried on singing the words of the anthem a capella once the music stopped.

Emotions were high. Tears welled up in the eyes of the players and the spectators. Half an hour later, they were in full flow. Germany eviscerated the hosts, in one of the most shocking sporting results of all time. They were 5-0 up at half-time and 7-1 up by the final whistle, as a shellshocked nation watched on in horror. The ghosts of 1950 were alive and well. Brazil simply fell to pieces, in front of a home crowd, again.

The sense of incredulity experienced by millions watching at home was echoed on the pitch. Here's Germany midfielder Mesut Ozil talking to *Sport* a few months later: 'After 25 minutes, I took a deep breath. I thought to myself: is this really happening? We were playing Brazil, in Brazil, and they were having a good tournament like us. We were expecting a really tough game. How could we be 3-0, 4-0 up?'

Brazil's team of hardened, successful professionals simply collapsed under the immense pressure of the situation. 'It was probably the lowest point of every single one of the Brazilian players involved and I don't think I exaggerate when I say we will probably have to answer questions about that game for the rest of our lives,' said Manchester City midfielder Fernandinho, who played for Brazil in that game, in an interview with the *Guardian*. 'We will need to learn to live with that.

'I don't think there is one simple answer for that result,' he continued. '. . . But we have to admit that we simply froze during those six minutes. And that killed the game for us. I am sure we could pinpoint other factors, but I have never watched a replay of that game and I don't think I ever will.

'The buck stopped with the players and on that night we didn't have the mental strength to recover from the shock of conceding an early goal. If anything, I just think we were not prepared to lose.'

The way experts crack under pressure is one of the most studied topics in sports psychology, and one of the areas in which practitioners really get the chance to prove their worth. Choking, bottling it, or whatever you want to call it, isn't just confined to stunning collapses like Brazil's – it can be individual moments of madness, or simply athletes performing below their capabilities in pressure situations.

Only experts have the capacity to choke. 'Choking is suboptimal performance, not just poor performance,' writes Sian Beilock, one of the leading researchers in this area, in her book aptly titled *Choke*. 'We all have performance ups and downs, but choking occurs when performers perceive a situation to be highly stressful and, because of the stress, they screw up. Choking is most noticeable when an opportunity to win is squandered, perhaps because this is when the pressure to excel is at its highest. Choking is not random.'

The names of the chokers are writ large in the sporting annals: Greg Norman turning a six-shot lead into a five-shot defeat against Nick Faldo at the 1996 Masters; Jimmy White missing a black off the spot in the 1994 World Snooker final; almost every England penalty shoot-out at a major international tournament. In each case, well-trained brains simply couldn't handle the pressure.

Home Disadvantage

We tend to think of home advantage as one of the immutable laws of sport. It is clear to see in results across a range of sports: it works out at around 60 per cent in baseball, around 70 per cent in basketball and around 60 per cent in football. You only have to look at the medal tables for home Olympics to see how much better the host country does than in previous or subsequent Games.

But it doesn't always work that way, as in Brazil's case in the 1950 and 2014 World Cups, or for dozens of Brits at Wimbledon until Andy Murray came along. With a feverish crowd at their backs, players are supposed to be able to give that little bit extra, while the opposition are cowed and intimidated. But what if players are able to win at home *despite* the support of the home crowd and not because of it?

In the 1980s, a team of psychologists led by Roy Baumeister tried to find out the effect of a supportive crowd on the execution of skill, separate from the other variables that could cause a home advantage, such as greater familiarity with the conditions or having less distance to travel than the opposition before the game. They trawled through the archives of championship games in Major League Baseball. These games are played as a series – seven matches split home and away with the winner of the series being the first to reach four wins. You would expect home advantage to play a large part in determining success in these situations, but when Baumeister looked at games where the home team was just one more victory away from clinching the series, he found that they lost almost two-thirds of the time.

The home disadvantage effect has been observed in other sports, from golfers playing on their home course, to ice hockey teams vying for the Stanley Cup in front of their own fans. The 2012 Champions League final is another example. Chelsea came up shock winners on penalties against Bayern Munich, in Munich, echoing the final of 1984 when Liverpool beat Roma on penalties in Rome.

Brazil's 7-1 World Cup thrashing was probably a perfect storm of pressure. They had been criticised early on in the tournament, had lacked their traditional fluidity, and faced a tough match against a formidable opponent, with the ghost of Barbosa never far away. They were also without their star player, who had been instrumental in getting them to that stage. Is it any wonder that a demanding crowd turned into a disadvantage?

Even having just one person standing in the room watching you can make you perform worse, as Baumeister found out when he asked people to play a computer game called *Sky Jinks*. Originally released in 1982 for the Atari 2600, it's typical of games of that era – primary colours and a simple control scheme masking surprising difficulty. Players control a small plane with a joystick and have to pilot it through an obstacle course as quickly as they can. It's a test of co-ordination and concentration, like sport.

Baumeister gave people plenty of practice at the game, and waited until they were really good at it. Then, he introduced a stranger to stand in the room and act as if either supportive or uninterested. The players did worse in front of a supportive audience than they did in front of a neutral audience. You may have experienced this yourself: ever noticed how your ability to type seems to stutter if someone is standing over you watching?

People are also more likely to choke when there's something at stake, even if it's just a small amount of cash, as Baumeister discovered when he offered participants $3 if they could match their previous performances in a final run-through of *Sky Jinks* at the end of the first experiment. Most of them couldn't, because of the added pressure.

The same thing has been observed in sport. When a free throw in the last five minutes of an NBA game has the potential to draw their team level, players are 7 per cent less likely to score.

When the stakes are higher, the pressure is higher, and performance suffers. In one study at Cambridge University, participants had their brain activity scanned with fMRI while they played a computer game similar to *Pac-Man*. Some were offered a 50p reward every time they successfully caught a grey dot moving around a maze, while others were offered a £5 reward.

Those offered the bigger reward did worse. Instead of sharpening their focus, the extra cash caused them to miss turnings in the maze and catch the dot fewer times overall. Their brains also behaved differently: fMRI analysis found that poor performance was correlated with increased activity in an area of the brain called the ventral striatum, which is thought to be involved in processing risk and reward.

In this case, the extra cash meant that the brain's reward system was too active, and it interfered with the players' ability to perform.

Another fMRI study at Caltech also offered participants a cash reward for a task requiring hand-eye co-ordination, with rewards ranging from \$0 to \$100. They found that performances improved as the cash on offer increased, but only up to a certain point. Above that level, performance fell sharply, as activity in the ventral striatum intensified. The researchers concluded that performances suffered because of loss aversion – participants were worried about losing a potential reward, and this caused their performance to deteriorate.

So whether it's the prospect of winning a medal or tying the game for your team, the size of the reward on offer or the potential magnitude of looming failure can cause athletes' performances to worsen under pressure. In Brazil's case it was probably a bit of both: the opportunity to reach the World Cup final at home and put the demons of 1950 to rest, on top of the potential shame of failure, wreaked havoc with the players' reward systems. The increased activity in the ventral striatum was combined with an amygdala hijack, and the impaired function of the prefrontal cortex under stress meant the players were unable to keep their emotions in check. They choked, spectacularly.

Would it have all been different if Neymar had been fit? Maybe not. As the talisman of the team, there was extra pressure on his young shoulders, and research suggests the added burden may have made him more likely to choke.

Norwegian Dr Geir Jordet has worked as a penalty shoot-out consultant for the Dutch national team, another side with a famously bad historic record from the spot. He's made an extensive study of the art of scoring from 12 yards, including going through the archives to watch every penalty shoot-out ever conducted in the World Cup, European Championships and Champions League. He then compared the record of players with a high public status, those who had finished in the top three in awards such as FIFA Player of the Year or South American Footballer of the Year. What he found was surprising. Publicly appreciated superstars such as Cristiano Ronaldo or Lionel Messi are more likely, on average, to miss penalties than their less individually decorated counterparts. Messi's penalty record is particularly bad. As of October 2015, he'd missed 17 out of 81 career spot kicks.

Croatia's penalty shoot-out against Turkey in the quarter-finals of Euro 2008 is another example. I happened to be watching the game with friends in a pizza restaurant near Umag on Croatia's Istrian coast. It wasn't a great game; we were really only waiting for the thunderstorms to stop so we could walk back to our rented villa. Then, towards the end of extra time, things started to get pretty stormy.

Croatian playmaker Luka Modric had the ball deep in the Turkish half, but his back was to goal and he was in no real position of threat until Turkey's ponytailed keeper Rustu Recber suffered a rush of blood to the head (or an amygdala hijack) and charged off his line to try to close him down. Having vacated his line, Rustu watched in horror as the ball was lobbed into the centre, and headed past his scrambling attempt to recover and into the net. The celebrations were wild, both in the stadium in Switzerland and in our little restaurant, as Croatia thought they were going through, but the cheers were soon cut short.

Turkey equalised with the last kick of the game to set up a penalty shoot-out – and it was star player Modric up first. 'When I saw Luka Modric walking to the penalty spot, I knew he was going to miss,' said Jordet, who had just submitted his paper and must have been watching the shoot-out with a heightened interest even greater than our waiter's. 'The Croatian team had just been given a psychological knockout blow by the Turks but, more importantly, Modric is the biggest star in the Croatian team and that status increases the chance of failure. If expectations are higher, you are more likely to miss.'

The theory is that because these players are held in such high esteem by fans, they've got much more to lose if they do miss, adding extra pressure to an already difficult task. The more players have to lose, the worse they perform. According to Jordet, 'If a penalty can bring a team an instant win, 92 per cent of the time the shot is on target. If, however, missing will bring the team instant defeat, only 62 per cent of the shots will produce a goal.'

Paralysis By Analysis

Monte Carlo is a ridiculous place, especially over a race weekend. I've been lucky enough to make the trip to the Monaco Grand Prix once, where I watched the cars negotiate the tight right-hand turn known as 'Casino' from the balcony of said casino, with slot machines flashing in the background. There was a copy of a magazine called *Yacht Investor* on the bar, which says it all really.

The circuit is legendary. It's tight, twisty and dangerous. Former F1 champion Nelson Piquet has likened it to riding a bicycle around your living room. It requires incredible focus and concentration, as drivers are just inches from disaster, but it remains the race that they want to win more than anything, regardless of what level they're racing at.

That was certainly the case for Sam Bird, one of motorsport's journeymen. Born in Roehampton, in south-west London, the 29-year-old has worked his way up through the confusing maze of junior formulae without ever quite getting the chance to make it into Formula 1, where securing a seat depends as much on your financial muscle as your ability behind the wheel. He has the short stature of a racing driver, and measures his words carefully.

In 2011, Bird was racing in GP2, a support series just below F1, which follows some of the same calendar and uses some of the same tracks. He had enjoyed a good start to the season, picking up three podiums from the first four races, and he looked to be in strong shape for another when he was promoted to pole position in Monaco after qualifying.

It's notoriously difficult to overtake in Monte Carlo's narrow streets, so being on pole automatically makes you the favourite to win the race. But not for Bird, who let the prestige and the pressure get to him. 'Emotional pressure has affected my results,' he told me. 'I qualified in pole position in Monaco in 2011 and I let the stress of that get to me so much that I stalled at the start.'

It was a disaster. By the time the cars had climbed the short hill to St Devote, the first corner, Bird had gone from first to last. He managed to battle back to 11th before being forced into retirement on lap 31 after twice making contact with his teammate.

'I put so much pressure on myself to get to the first corner first,' he recalls. 'I went round and round and round in my head – you have to get off the line, you have to get off the line, you have to get into the first corner first, you have to do a brilliant start, and I overanalysed the start, I overthought it, tried to do something far too complicated and stalled the car.'

Psychologists call this 'explicit monitoring' or 'paralysis by analysis'. The theory came out of Roy Baumeister's work with *Sky Jinks*, and is widely accepted as one of the main reasons that athletes sometimes fail to perform under pressure. In chapter two we looked at how athletes are able to perform extraordinary feats of co-ordination by making complicated movements automatic. Paralysis by analysis happens when, because of pressure or other external forces, they start consciously paying attention to actions that should be instinctive.

In 2003, a group of Dutch researchers asked people to tackle a climbing wall, starting either low on the wall as normal or higher up. They found that those who started higher up the wall reported greater levels of anxiety, unsurprisingly, that their heart rates were higher and that they showed higher levels of muscle fatigue. What's interesting is that, as they climbed these identical routes at different heights, the climbers further up the wall were much less fluent in their movements; because of the pressure of being higher up the wall, they were thinking about what they were doing too much, and their movements slowed down.

When there's a big reward on offer, or a big penalty for failure, or even when there's a supportive audience willing them to succeed, athletes start thinking too much about what they're doing, and that often spells disaster.

In her youth, Sian Beilock played football and was a promising goalkeeper. She has first-hand experience of choking under pressure, from a state-wide tournament where recruiters were invited to watch. 'I didn't make the saves I should have made,' she has said. 'I knew all eyes were on me, and so I started thinking way too much about aspects of my performance that should have been left on autopilot.'

Nowadays, Beilock is a professor of psychology at the University of Chicago, and one of the world's experts on why athletes choke. She has collected evidence in support of the paralysis by analysis theory in a couple of neat studies that show how asking athletes to think about what they're doing is actually much more detrimental to their performance than distracting them with something else.

In one study, she asked expert and novice footballers to dribble through a slalom course using either their dominant or weaker foot. In the 'skill-focused' part of the test, the participants were asked to pay attention to whether they were kicking the ball with the inside or outside of their foot (a successful dribbling motion requires both), and to say whether they'd just touched it with the inside or outside when a tone was played. In the 'dual-task' condition, they were given a target word and a tape of random words was played while they dribbled. They had to repeat the target word when they heard it.

The experienced athletes took several seconds longer to make it through the course when they were asked to pay attention to their movements, compared to when they were simply asked to shout out the target word. This effect did not exist for the novices, and it disappeared when the experts used their weaker foot. The skill in these cases had not yet become automatic and was still under conscious control, so forcing them to think about it didn't make a difference because they were already thinking about it.

Professor Rob Gray at Arizona State University found a similar phenomenon with college baseball players. He put them in a batting cage and asked them to listen out for a tone while they faced pitches, and report whether they had heard a high tone or a low tone. This had no effect on their hitting ability. He also asked them to listen for the tone and monitor what point in their swing they were at when it sounded. As in the footballers, explicitly monitoring their performance in this way made them much worse; their movements became less fluid, their swings got slower and choppier. Something that should have been chunked and automatic came under conscious control, and there wasn't enough working memory available to perform.

A study by a group based in London looked at what happens in the brain when people are asked to pay attention to a skill they've already learnt. The prefrontal cortex is heavily involved in the learning of new skills, but it recedes into the background as they become more automatic. But when people or athletes start paying attention to those well-honed skills, it seizes control again (with the left hemisphere particularly culpable), as movements become slow and less fluent.

Fernandinho must have controlled a football perfectly hundreds of thousands of times in his life. But, at 3-0 down against Germany in a World Cup semi-final, something went wrong as he received a pass midway inside his own half with his back to goal. His touch was heavy, clunky. The ball span a yard away off his foot, was poached by an onrushing Toni Kroos and, seconds later, it was in the back of the net – 4-0 to the Germans. When the ball was coming towards Fernandinho, with his team already 3-0 down in front of 74,000 fans and a German midfielder closing in, he may have been paying too much attention to the movements he needed to make to control the ball properly, telling himself he *had* to get a good touch. So, instead of the automatic part of his brain weighing up all the variables he needed to take into account and making the correct movement, his prefrontal cortex seized control and he reverted to the ponderous, slower and less accurate movements of the novice performer.

When you're learning a skill, you piece it together from smaller chunks. Learning to drive, for example, is a process of working the accelerator and clutch, as well as steering and finding the right gear. After a while it becomes automatic, but if you start paying attention to it, for example if you have to explain what you're doing to someone else, things can start to go wrong.

When the stakes are high, people start paying attention to things that should be automatic, and thousands of hours of practice can evaporate in an instant.

Jean van de Velde and The Cognichoke

Sport isn't just about running on autopilot – sometimes athletes have to make higher-level decisions. And sometimes, when they're under pressure, distracted or emotional, they make really bad decisions. Take golfer Jean van de Velde's infamous collapse at the Open in 1999. *Sports Illustrated* describe it like this: 'Standing on the tee of the final hole on Sunday, Van de Velde had a three-stroke lead. Twenty excruciating minutes later he was bent over a six-foot putt, needing to hole it to get into a playoff ... To get from point A to point B the Frenchman had hit the wrong club off the tee, chosen an even worse club from the rough for his second shot, bruised a grandstand, wound up barefoot in a burn and pitched into a greenside bunker, performing with such consistent disregard for his position that old-timers were reminded of Wrong-Way Corrigan, the aviator of the '30s who set off from New York for Los Angeles and flew instead to Ireland.'

This is a different kind of choking entirely. It's not paralysis by analysis, and actually it seems to happen for the exact opposite reason. Instead of paying too much attention to something that should be automatic, demands on working memory mean athletes aren't paying enough attention and therefore make errors of judgement, choosing the wrong pass, the wrong club, the wrong tactic. 'Sports aren't cognitively static,' Beilock told *Wired*. 'Situations change, and you need to track things and make decisions. You can't just not think. There's a whole skill involved in knowing not just what not to think about, but when to attend to things that need tending. You've got to be able to control what you're attending to.'

Earlier on, we looked at the limited capacity of working memory. The theory is that under stress or emotional pressure, working memory can become overloaded with negative thoughts, so when athletes have to make higher-level decisions about what club to use, for example, or how to play a particular point in tennis, they don't have the mental resources available to properly reason through the options as they would normally.

Writing in *Wired*, science journalist David Dobbs calls this kind of choke a 'cognichoke' – a disruption of higher-level decision-making that has more in common with the way people choke in job interviews or exams. Researchers at the University of Pennsylvania scanned people's brains while they did a subtraction task which asked them to subtract 13 from a four-digit number, and go faster and faster as they did so. As things sped up, they found increased blood flow to regions such as the right prefrontal cortex, which is associated with negative emotions. They also found that the increased blood flow to this area led to decreased blood flow to the left prefrontal cortex – the area of the brain involved in thinking and verbal reasoning. This effect lasts for a while. Even after the stressful situation is over, the effects of depleted resources can still impact on decision-making. Stress uses up mental bandwidth.

It's an interesting conundrum. Most sports require both a high level of automaticity for the execution of well-learnt motor skills, but also a degree of higher-level thinking so that athletes know when to execute which skills, and can take into account the wider situation in the game. These systems run in parallel, and both have their susceptibilities. To avoid choking under pressure, athletes need to be able to not focus on their precise physical movements in order to prevent paralysis by analysis, but they also need to be able to block out negative thoughts which could use up the working memory resources they need to make higher-level decisions.

To employ the terms used by Dr Steve Peters: when the Human takes over, rational thoughts interfere with things that should be left automatic and it's paralysis by analysis, but when the Chimp seizes control worries take up working memory, resulting in a cognichoke. As Dobbs puts it, athletes need to understand what to distract themselves from (physical mechanics) and what not to get distracted from (the score, the time left in the game).

The Yips

Steven Finn is annoyed. We're sitting in a meeting room overlooking Trent Bridge cricket ground a couple of days before the Fourth Test between England and Australia in the summer of 2015, and I've just brought up the 'Y' word. The lanky fast bowler had returned to the England side for the first time since being sent home from their tour of Australia in the winter of 2013/14 because of problems with his bowling action. His selection proved pivotal in the Third Test – he redeemed himself by taking eight wickets as England defied expectations to clinch a victory that helped them seal the Ashes. I ask him what had gone wrong with his bowling during his time in the wilderness: was it paralysis by analysis?

'The thing is, when you're not feeling in rhythm as a bowler, you search for things,' he tells me. 'You search for a reason for why you're not in rhythm. Sometimes it might be because the ground's funny or sometimes it might be because something with your action is awry. I was looking for a golden nugget of information that was going to set me free and make me into the bowler that I knew I was capable of being. But there's no such thing, and when you're practising day in, day out and you're grooving habits, you have to unravel them and make them better. There's no one bit of information that's just going to make it better. So it was important that I took a little bit of time off to reassess where I was at, and then I just attacked it from there really.'

Sometimes, athletes lose their ability to perform the simplest of tasks and never recover. This affliction has many names. When five-time world darts champion Eric Bristow gradually lost the ability to release the projectile properly, he dubbed it 'dartitis'. It has also been called 'cueitis' in snooker, 'flinching' in shooting and 'target panic' in archery. Baseball fans might know it as 'the creature', 'the monster' or 'Steve Sax syndrome', after the former LA Dodgers second baseman who suddenly lost the ability to make routine throws. But this affliction is most commonly referred to as 'the yips', and it can affect performers in all manner of sports, but particularly in golf, baseball and cricket. It has ruined careers, which might explain why Finn baulks at applying it to his situation.

'See, it annoys me when people use that word because "the yips" are when you can't let go of the ball, you can't run up to the crease, you can't do anything,' he says. 'I've got video footage of a net that I had the day before I left Australia where I bowled every single ball fine; it's just my rhythm was just out and my mechanics were a bit messed up. So it frustrates me and annoys me when people use that word, because it's just totally not true and it's actually quite an offensive word to use – particularly when you're talking about a bowler, because it means that they've completely lost it.'

Scott Boswell is a YouTube sensation. The video he stars in has racked up over a million views. Unfortunately, it's called 'The Worst Over Ever?' and depicts an agonising spell which effectively ended Boswell's career as a professional sportsman. In 2001, Leicestershire reached the final of the C&G Trophy – county cricket's equivalent of the League Cup. In the semi-final, the 26-year-old had secured the best figures of his career, taking four wickets for just 44 runs, and setting up the biggest game of his career so far. 'It was going to be one of the best days of my life,' he told the *Guardian* in a rare interview more than a decade on.

It took him 14 balls instead of six to complete his second over of the game. Six of his first eight balls were wides. Watching the footage is harrowing, like a waking nightmare, as Boswell retrieves the ball from his teammates and turns to try again, with little control over where it will end up. '[The batsman] looked as though he was 50 yards away,' remembered Boswell. 'He was like a tiny dot. I just couldn't see him. Then I bowled a wide and I heard the noise of the crowd. I bowled a second wide, and the noise got louder and louder and louder. I just couldn't let go of the ball. I wanted to get on with it, so I began to rush. The more I panicked, the more I rushed.'

It's thought that there are actually two causes for the yips, which are characterised by involuntary jerks, tremors and spasms. The type that likely affected Boswell is an extreme form of paralysis by analysis, where athletes are unable to stop focusing on their finer movements (generally called Type II yips). It's a cruel affliction because worrying about being unable to release the ball or make a putt properly only increases the likelihood of getting it wrong. It's different from choking because it's enduring, and often has a trigger that's external to sport.

Sports psychologist Dr Mark Bawden has worked with the England and Wales Cricket Board (ECB) and the English Institute of Sport to help athletes with the yips. 'I think it's very similar to a phobia,' he tells me. 'Something like a sports performance phobia, where someone has experienced a significant event either in the performance itself or outside of the performance arena. Basically people go into that kind of fight, flight, freeze scenario and it becomes an ongoing, permanent thing.'

He thinks it's qualitatively different from choking under pressure – that pressure magnifies but doesn't cause the yips. 'Where it gets confusing is if you take an example like Scott Boswell, although it started off as a choking experience – bowling a wide ball – it ended up being a fairly horrific experience where he feels like he's stuck in front of a lot of people. As a result of that it becomes almost phobic, and then the next time he comes into bowl his brain is on high alert and looking for similar cues – just a little bit of evidence that the same thing is going to happen again, and it does.'

Bawden thinks people who are more self-conscious are more prone to the yips, and that they are especially common among bowlers in cricket because of the nature of the sport. If they bowl a wide or a no-ball, they have to repeat the delivery until they get it right – literally becoming trapped in a never-ending cycle of failure.

So while this type of yips is simply an extreme, prolonged form of choking, perhaps exacerbated by underlying emotional trauma, the other form is something else entirely. In her unusual office at Arizona State University, Debbie Crews is trying to get to the bottom of it. Instead of the institutional carpet you might expect to find in a university building, her room has artificial turf. Two round holes have been cut into it and covered with sticky tape. It's a makeshift putting green, where Crews tests golfers with the yips to find out why and how it happens.

She has used a device called the CyberGlove, which has 17 different sensors to measure the movement of muscles in the hands and the fingers as golfers attempt to putt. In addition to that, she's built her own sensors which are placed on the wrist and lower forearm to track the activities of those muscles, and pick up on the rotation of the arm as the club comes through.

She has found that in some cases – probably about 7 to 10 per cent – the yips are caused by 'focal dystonia', a condition where nearby muscles co-contract, creating the spasms and jerks typical of the disorder. When athletes train, their brain changes because of neural plasticity; the more they use a particular muscle or group of muscles, the bigger the area of the brain that controls that part of the body gets. Focal dystonia is thought to happen when those areas of the brain start growing too large, and begin to run together and overlap. The brain loses its ability to selectively control muscle groups, the same way you might struggle to move your little toes independently of each other.

'I believe that's the theoretical framework that makes the most sense at this point,' says Crews when I speak to her on the phone from her office. 'It's the sensory input areas that tend to be disrupted in focal dystonia, or enlarged compared to what it should be, because they're skilled performers,' she says. 'That's then what affects the motor programme going to the muscles.'

That's what afflicted snooker player Stephen Hendry, a cruel twist for the beneficiary of one of the most famous choking incidents in UK sporting history – Jimmy White's missed black. 'On some shots I don't even get the cue through,' Hendry told the BBC after being knocked out of the UK Championship in 2010. 'It's so frustrating; it's like giving these guys a 50-point head start, it's horrendous. It's got gradually worse for 10 years.'

This is typical of Type I yips, or 'true yips' as Crews calls them. In contrast to Boswell's sudden attack, they develop gradually over a period of time. Type II yips are on the same spectrum as choking, simply a more severe version, but it's becoming clear that Type I yips are something entirely different, according to Crews. 'People clearly can choke, but they show no spasm or jerk, and the people who have a spasm or jerk don't necessarily choke – they just have no control over the motion.

'They're gonna yip in their living room, hitting a golf ball to a table leg with nobody looking and nobody cares if they hit it, they're still going to yip. But with almost everybody else it would never occur in that situation.'

This kind of yips tends to afflict athletes later on in their careers – Hendry, Bristow and golfer Tom Watson have all struggled with it in their twilight years. Crews told me that while the average age of onset across a range of studies into Type II yips varied from 31 to 56, the average years spent playing was between 20.9 and 31. Athletes spend years growing their motor maps so that they can perform with more precision, but it's when they get too big that the yips start to happen – the same way that in certain sports putting on too much muscle can actually be counterproductive.

Hendry continued: 'I think I need to phone Bernhard Langer to see how he got over the "yips" because that's what I have.' Golfer Langer got over the yips by taking advantage of neural plasticity, essentially retraining his brain by relearning the skill in a slightly different way and changing the sensory input. He developed a new type of grip, now named after him, where the right hand braces the shaft of the putter against the forearm of the left hand.

Relearning skills is a common form of treatment for all types of yips. 'Someone may have had a fairly horrific experience on the greens,' says Bawden, 'but by a simple change of technique the brain is almost tricked into doing something different and you can get around the problem very quickly.'

Other strategies include those adopted by golfer Johnny Miller, from painting a dab of red nail polish on the grip of his putter and focusing on that, to looking at the hole instead of the ball, or putting with his eyes closed. They all involve changing the sensory input to the brain, and therefore building new pathways within it. Crews has been able to help 'yippers' by giving golfers ski gloves to wear while they putt, so the club doesn't feel like a putter anymore, while the controversial belly putter has also aided some. In golf, Bawden has found he can eliminate the yips temporarily in some cases when he replaces the golf ball with a tennis ball.

'The yips are getting a lot more prevalent in chipping right now, and there are fewer options to change it than with putting,' says Crews. 'One thing that has been very successful is separating the hands so that they don't touch. When you change it from a uni-manual task to a bi-manual task, the brain receives it very differently and that can be very effective for chipping.'

Another thing that could help is taking advantage of the brain's plasticity and essentially starting from scratch, allowing the neural maps to atrophy and then rebuilding them. Studies of people with writer's cramp and musicians with focal dystonia have found that stabilising the muscles with a brace for a period of time, and then training them afterwards with writing tasks or ball exercises, could help reduce the yips.

Direct electrical stimulation of the motor cortex could also be productive, if the exact location of the areas controlling problem muscles could be pinpointed within the brain. A few sessions of electrical stimulation have been found to have a positive impact on people with musician's cramp or writer's cramp, both forms of focal dystonia, like Type II yips.

One of the things that Crews and others have found with their EMG devices is that signs of the yips can be found in the muscles before the player is even aware of them, small muscle twitches that aren't intense enough to cause the spasms or affect performance yet. She believes that players will soon start seeking out preventative treatment at an earlier stage, before the yips become a problem, although at heart she believes a flexible approach to sport is key and talk of a 'cure' is far-fetched.

'I've seen it travel from the right hand to the left hand, back to the right hand – this is a tour player who has won on the tour with the yips,' she says. 'It isn't so much a matter of curing it or fixing it; my pitch is for them to learn to play with the yips and have multiple strategies. The people who come in and just want to beat it and find the one fix or cure, to me that's part of the problem that got them the yips – the idea that there's one perfect way they have to move in order to get successful.'

Crews believes that flexibility of movement is key to avoiding the yips – having multiple strategies for getting the ball from point A to point B – which makes sense from a neurological point of view too, in terms of those enlarged motor maps. 'You putt the ball in many different ways,' she says. 'You draw it in, you fade it in. They would be better off if we would encourage them to be creative instead of very mechanical.'

The yips remain rare. But everyone, whether they're an athlete or not, will have felt their performances deteriorate under pressure and seen at first hand the effects of an amygdala hijack that we've covered in this chapter. But, as we'll see in the next, athletes are using a whole range of new techniques and technologies to help them perform under pressure, and they're techniques that can help you too.

CHAPTER SEVEN

TIGER WOODS AND THE POWER OF PRESSURE

Earl Woods was a talented athlete in his own right – he'd won a baseball scholarship to Kansas State University – but when watching his son Tiger practising on the golf course he would turn into the clumsiest man alive. Woods senior would drop golf bags, jingle change in his pocket, cough as his son pulled his club back for drives, and roll balls across his line of sight when he was going for putts. This is a form of 'pressure training', which is just one of the methods athletes can use to fight choking that we'll look at in this chapter.

'I really don't think we are born being able to thrive or succeed versus fail under pressure,' said Sian Beilock in a documentary broadcast on BBC Radio 4. 'I think the goal and the reason that some people are able to perform well is because they've developed the tools, and I would argue largely psychological tools so that in the moment they can put their best foot forward.'

Over the last few years, psychologists have been using what they've learnt about how the brain contributes to athletic performance to develop new training techniques and strategies to eliminate poor performance under stress. There are ways of training the brain to be more resilient to pressure.

There are a number of examples in Beilock's book *Choke* of the power of pressure training. Southern Utah's college basketball team were 217th in the national free-throw rankings when their coach Roger Reid introduced random free-throw drills during training. Players would have to sprint around the court if they missed. They rose up the rankings to first.

In the run-up to the London 2012 Olympics, the English Institute of Sport's head of psychology, Pete Lindsay, worked with judo players to simulate the pressure of performing. 'In order to recreate pressure, we might manipulate the demands the environment places on a player,' he said. This involves things such as making the fighting area smaller, or pre-fatiguing players so they get practice of fighting under physical duress.

As well as preparing athletes for emotional and physical stress, pressure training can directly fight paralysis by analysis, and stop athletes paying too much attention to well-learnt skills. One study found that filming golfers during their practice sessions and telling them that the video would be watched by a golf coach later can make them perform better in a subsequent pressure-filled competition. They get used to being watched.

Paralysis by analysis happens when the prefrontal cortex grabs the controls of processes that should be automatic. One way to stop it from doing that is to give it something else to do. After Beilock's career as a goalkeeper, she moved on to lacrosse at college, where she found that she had better luck getting the ball at face-offs if she sang to herself to stop herself from thinking too much.

When athletes pay attention to skills they've already learnt, it's the brain's left hemisphere that is doing the overthinking. A team of German researchers were able to improve performance under pressure by asking athletes to squeeze a ball in their left hand as they performed their skill. Because the left side of the body is controlled by the right hemisphere of the brain (and vice versa), doing this draws neural resources like glucose and oxygen away from the interfering left hemisphere and reduces its negative influence on automatic processes.

In football, the test the researchers used to test performance under pressure was, inevitably, penalty kicks. First, 30 semi-pro players took practice shots to determine their base level of performance. Then the following day they did the same again in front of a crowd of 300 students waiting to watch a match on television. The players who took penalties as normal missed more shots than they had the day before, while the players who squeezed a small ball in their left hand managed to maintain their performance levels. The same pattern of results was found with judo experts who were told that their kicking practice was going to be videotaped and evaluated by top coaches. Those who squeezed a ball in their left hand performed better. Badminton shuns balls, and so did the badminton players in a third experiment. Players who simply clenched their left hand during play regularly beat players who weren't using this technique when they competed in front of their coaches.

After Rory McIlroy's collapse at the 2011 Masters (a classic choke, he said afterwards that he was 'trying to be too focused, too perfect'), he started working with ex-pro Dave Stockton, who was renowned during his playing days for being one of the game's best putters. Stockton, who wrote a book called *Unconscious Putting*, focused on just that, and tried to get McIlroy to stop thinking about what he was doing with his body. 'The work that I've done with Dave Stockton has been more about how to approach a putt, not focusing on technique, so much more like green reading, your routine, and everything like that,' said McIlroy.

'If I have any sort of technical thing in my thought, in my stroke, it would just be to keep the back of my left hand going towards the target, and that's all we really worked on. It seemed to work.'

That's an example of a focus cue, which gives the athlete something specific to concentrate on so they're not obsessing over their action. They've been used to great success across a range of sports. Tennis coaches sometimes ask players to exhale or say the word 'hit' when they strike the ball. The grunting you sometimes hear during tennis matches, that's a focus cue too.

Legendary golfer Jack Nicklaus would reportedly think about his little toe during his swing; while, before an attempted penalty or conversion, England rugby player Jonny Wilkinson would focus intently on both the precise point of the ball he wanted to make contact with and a person in the crowd who was sitting in line with the trajectory of the kick he was about to attempt.

Gabriele Wulf and colleagues at the University of Nevada found that simply asking people to focus their attention externally rather than internally was a great way of improving their performance. Slalom skiers learnt faster on a simulator if they focused on a marked spot in front of them, while golfers who focused on the swing of the club rather than their arms were 20 per cent more accurate. Novice swimmers who concentrated on the movement of the water around their limbs started to move with the grace of experts, while experts' performance declined when they focused on their limbs.

The key is to give your prefrontal cortex something else to think about to stop it interfering. In certain situations, performing under pressure is all about getting your head out of the game.

There's an App For That

At the GlaxoSmithKline Human Performance Lab, I get a chance to try out one of the tests researchers are using to measure how an athlete's brain speed changes when they're exposed to various pressures. 'We're using simple iPad-based tools to look at fundamental cognitive processing and how that changes with environmental stressors,' says the lab's cognitive lead Dr Barry O'Neill. 'We are looking at the impact of where they play, where they train, their environmental conditions and how all that impacts cognitive function. That can give us a read on whether they're ready to train and compete.'

After O'Neill explains the task, I put on headphones and get going. The first test is simple: I have to tap a large circle in the centre of the screen as quickly as I can whenever it turns green. In another, circles appear randomly across the screen, one at a time, and I have to tap the green ones and avoid the red ones while a voice in the headphones tries to distract me by saying 'stop' or 'go' at inappropriate moments. The final group of tests involves a ring of circles, with an arrow in the centre. I have to tap the circle that the arrow is pointing towards, as long as it's the right colour, unless the voice in the headphones tells me otherwise.

Part of the rationale behind cognitive training tools is to make high-speed decision-making more resilient. 'We essentially increase the automaticity of high-speed decision-making to try and require as little of the bandwidth of the brain as possible,' says Jason Sada, whose company Axon Sports develops such tools. 'We know we're not going to eliminate emotional issues, but when they occur the brain has some extra bandwidth to deal with it. Ideally high-speed decision-making is unaffected and you can still make high-speed accurate decisions under an emotional load or with distractions.

'There are distractions that are relevant, and distractions that are irrelevant,' he continues. 'A coach yelling out what play to run is no question a distraction from playing, but it is extremely relevant. You have to listen to it. It is critical to your performance on the pitch. Whereas an opposing player talking to you is an irrelevant distraction ... although I suppose it depends on what he's saying! The same things exist physically. If you're injured or fatigued, your brain is allocating bandwidth to handling the situation with your body so it's taking away resources from decision-making.

'We have tasks that simulate relevant and irrelevant visual and auditory distractions,' Sada explains. I'm sceptical about how well this will work, but in a small room, with the headphones turned up loud in my ears, the auditory stimuli used by the HPL to elicit a feeling of stress do have an effect. The soundtrack includes a loud heartbeat, which increases during certain moments, as well as loud beeps and other distractions thrown in as well. 'If it was one constant sound your brain is quite good at filtering that out,' says O'Neill. 'For example, if you sit in an office with the AC going in the background, people tend not to hear it because your brain decides it's not really important. But when you present your brain with novel stimuli it's got to attribute some bandwidth to figure it out, and that's taking away the bandwidth from the task.'

It is harder to simulate emotional pressure. How can you possibly recreate the pressure of performing in front of thousands of spectators, with your life's work on the line in one moment? 'It's one of hardest things in the world,' says Sada. 'Every individual is unique and things that might trigger me emotionally might not trigger you. And things that might be significantly "de-focusing" to me might not be "de-focusing" to you.'

The emotional load on the test I try simply penalises you five times more heavily for a wrong answer. It works on me, as I make several mistakes in quick succession when under this condition. 'So far this is the best thing we've come up with,' says O'Neill. 'Because athletes are quite competitive by nature, and you have guys doing this in squad settings, they know their mates are gonna laugh at them if they blow up on these tasks.'

At the end of the battery of iPad tests, I'm given an average of my score across the different tasks with different auditory, visual and emotional distractions. I record an average of 0.755 seconds – marginally slower than Olympic triathlete Alistair Brownlee (0.748 seconds). I am, however, over 100 milliseconds slower than former F1 world champion Jenson Button, who scored one of the best times ever recorded in the HPL (0.643 seconds).

'These are components which may not differ massively between athletes and normal people,' says O'Neill. 'We didn't necessarily expect Jenson to be faster but it turned out he was significantly faster. He seemed to buck the trend with regards to the speed/accuracy trade-off. Usually what happens is that the faster you are, the less accurate you are, but it seemed like Jenson didn't have that trade-off – he was able to be both fast and accurate.'

Bad Robots

Australian cricket has a problem. English cricket too. Young batsmen coming through are finding it hard to play against really fast bowling. Trained in nets on bowling machines, these youngsters don't have enough experience of picking up the visual cues from the movement of the bowler's body. They have been very effectively trained on late detection of the ball's flight, but when the ball goes over a certain speed, that isn't enough.

That is Joan Vickers' warning. She is sceptical of tools designed to artificially boost a player's experience. 'Use ball machines a little bit,' she says. 'But you can use them way too much and basically destroy the skills of your hitters, and anyone with an interceptive timing skill.' Perhaps acknowledging this drawback of traditional bowling machines, the ECB recently ordered 20 of a new version which incorporates a large screen into a bowling machine set-up, so you can, for example, have a life-size Mitchell Johnson running towards you before the ball gets delivered.

Vickers' 'decision-training model' is all about structuring training in the right way, to avoid situations like the above and help ward off the choke. 'We now know that what happens with behavioural training is that athletes are put into mindless repetition over and over again,' says Vickers. 'They become mindless, and their bodies go through the motions. The big result of this is that when they are put under pressure, they don't have any training to handle unexpected events because they've never been exposed to unexpected events in their training.'

Her decision-training model, like Michel Bruyninckx's overload training, emphasises flexibility and novelty; it wants to prepare athletes for any possible eventuality and stop them from getting stuck in a rut. It has been implemented by Canada's Winter Olympics teams over the last 20 years.

'Block training is really one of the reasons that athletes choke,' says Vickers. 'You need to take those points of performance failure and you need to simulate them in practices, and what that does is change the brain – completely rewires it to develop these very rich neural networks that simply say, "I've seen this situation before thank you very much, I know exactly what to do."'

On his website, Daniel Coyle (the author of *The Talent Code*) highlights one example: an astonishing catch by Odell Beckham Jr, a wide receiver for the New York Giants. In a Sunday night game against the Dallas Cowboys in October 2014, Beckham Jr leapt into the air near the right corner of the field, extending one arm to pluck a pass from the sky with just his fingertips, despite interference from a tackler. He even managed to land in bounds to score a touchdown. A couple of months later, the jersey he was wearing when he made 'The Catch' was put on display in the Pro Football Hall of Fame, which should give you some idea of how outstanding it was.

It loses some of its mystical quality, although I think it becomes even more remarkable, when you watch some footage of the warm-ups before the game. There's Beckham Jr, Beats headphones on, practising catches in the end zone with one hand, the other pinned at his side, building up experience of guiding the ball safely to his chest with minimal contact, while on the stretch.

Coyle calls this 'high-leverage practice', and it's something good coaches and players have always done to help their players' performance under stressful conditions. But now they're getting a helping hand from researchers tapping into how the brain learns, and how practice can be tailored to cater to it.

When Less Is More

Teachers beware – here's a snide comeback for any pupil who ever gets snapped at to concentrate during a lesson. There's some evidence that, in certain situations, people learn better when they're not paying attention. Psychologists at Louisiana State University found that adults were better at learning a new language (in this case, a modified version of American Sign Language) when they were not paying too much attention to what they were being taught.

They showed college students a video that taught them how to sign simple sentences such as 'You help me' and 'I help you'. Some students watched the video on its own, while others watched but at the same time had to complete a task where a number of high-pitched tones played and they had to count them. Later on, the distracted students were better at combining the signs they'd learnt into new combinations. Because their working memory was being taxed by counting the tones, they couldn't hold everything in their head at once, so they learnt individual signs rather than whole sentences.

There's some debate among those designing cognitive training tools for sport about whether implicit learning like this is better than explicit learning. It echoes the debate in visualisation over whether it's better to use imagery from your own point of view, or of yourself in the third person. Interestingly, it seems that athletes in judged sports are more likely to do the latter, as are American football players, who spend a lot of time studying playbooks which show their position relative to others.

Normally, when you learn a skill, it is processed first by the conscious parts of the brain before progressing to automatic control. Implicit learning goes straight to the subconscious parts of the brain. At the University of Queensland, Bruce Abernethy has conducted experiments with tennis players similar to the American Sign Language experiment above. 'We showed people lots of clips, but we didn't ask them to predict where the serve was going or say anything about particular cues,' he tells me. 'We simply asked them to try and estimate the speed of the serve from the clips they were seeing. What that does is it means you're forcing attention on exactly the same areas but you're allowing the implicit processes in the brain to understand the relationship between shoulder angle and racket angle without learning a particular rule that you need to remember consciously.'

Implicit is often better; it's why we're always more fluent in our native tongue than any language we've learnt at school. 'There are some phenomenal athletes in the animal kingdom that have never been able to write down or verbally instruct how they do these things, but they seem to acquire the skills pretty well,' says Abernethy. 'So the question is, can you construct a learning environment that's not reliant on words and not reliant so much on consciousness, but allows these things to be discovered in a very automatic way?'

Implicit learning is also more resistant to stress. 'The beauty is, if things are below the level of consciousness, they're not then likely to be interfered with by conscious processes,' Abernethy says. 'If you're going out to play your very first Test match as a batsman you've got all kinds of conscious stuff running through your head – what if I fail, my parents are here, the scoreboard. If you're depending on getting cues consciously all that stuff interferes. If, however, the batting process is controlled below the level of consciousness, it goes on unaffected by all these other deliberate kinds of activities. It's another reason why trying to find ways to do things implicitly and automatically is pretty critical if you're going to get some real gains.'

In practice, for Vickers at least, this means withdrawing feedback, having the coaches say very little, and letting the athletes figure things out for themselves. 'In the first few years we put it in place, it caused a backlash,' she tells me. 'Some people are feedback junkies – they're in sport so they can be reinforced every day. Some of our coaches were elite figure skating coaches. You had parents paying $150 an hour to have this top coach coach their child, and the coach wasn't saying anything, and we got a lot of comments. But if you start withdrawing feedback and deliberately create situations in training where people have to develop, there are brain changes in neural function and attention and decision-making.'

No We Can't

In the 1992 sports comedy film *White Men Can't Jump,* Woody Harrelson plays Billy Hoyle, a talented street basketball player in Venice, Los Angeles. He makes a living hustling other players who believe that he'll be inferior to them at basketball because of his race. He is skilled at disrupting his opponent's concentration, something that can play a large part in success in a number of sports, from sledging in cricket to 'icing the kicker' in American football.

These techniques aren't new, but psychology and neuroscience can give athletes a better understanding not only of how to stop themselves from choking, but also how to make their opponents do it more. Italian defender Marco Materazzi's comment to French talisman Zinedine Zidane in extra time of the 2006 World Cup final was a throwaway remark, but it triggered an amygdala hijack that got Zidane sent off and helped Italy win the tournament. In his autobiography, Uruguay and Barcelona striker Luis Suarez talks about how players will target him with late challenges early on in games to try to get a reaction out of him. Emotion can be exploited, as Germany discovered in the 7-1 crushing of Brazil. Here's their coach Joachim Low in Raphael Honigstein's *Das Reboot*: 'We met the Brazilians' deep emotions with stamina, calmness, clarity and insistence, and we coolly exploited their weaknesses. We knew that their defence would be disorganised if we attacked quickly.'

Even the slightest provocation can raise someone's heart rate just enough to alter their decision-making – enticing them into playing a shot they don't need to in cricket and getting out, or playing a hand they don't need to in poker and getting wiped out. Poker player Daniel Negreanu is an expert at this; it's helped him win more than $30m in prize money. The 42-year-old has stayed at the top of the game despite an influx of younger, more mathematically minded players, and he told me his secret. 'The more uncomfortable I make them, the better off I am,' he says. 'Against these young guys, I'll make them as uncomfortable as I feel like I need to, just to let them know that . . .' At this point he starts shouting. 'This is my turf, you are at my table and *you will be grilled!* It's my way of asserting dominance.'

A technique such as icing the kicker, whereby an opposing coach calls a time-out just before a kick is taken, works because it gives the kick-taker more time to think about what he's about to do, and more chance for paralysis by analysis. Playing faster is one of the techniques used to fight choking – this is one of the things that Rory McIlroy worked on with Dave Stockton when trying to improve his putting. 'People often said to me, "We think you're too quick on the greens,"' McIlroy said. 'But he [Stockton] thought the opposite. You're taking too much time, why are you taking three practice strokes? Don't take any practice strokes anymore. See the target, where I want to hit it, and just go with it.'

If you can prevent your opponent from playing at the pace they want to, and force them to think, it can cause them to overthink. This is why you see goalkeepers arguing with referees long after penalties have been awarded – they know there's no chance of them being rescinded, they just want enough time to plant the seeds of the choke in the kick-taker's mind. A study of crucial field goal kicks in the 2002 and 2003 NFL seasons found that icing the kicker does seem to work.

Another tip for the trash talkers from neuroscience and Beilock's research: telling someone not to mess something up makes them more likely to do so. Even simply reminding them of certain negative characteristics of their team or any group they belong to could have a similar effect.

A few months before Barack Obama accepted the nomination to be the Democratic Party's presidential candidate in 2008, a group of 500 Americans took a test called the GRE (Graduate Record Examination).

This is normally used as an entry test for admission to graduate school, but in this case there was nothing riding on it – the test-takers had simply volunteered for a study. The results bore out a pattern seen across America: black test-takers did significantly worse on the test than their white counterparts, despite being matched for education level.

When the same test was given again immediately after Obama's inauguration later that year, the gap between the races had disappeared. This phenomenon is called stereotype threat, and it has been observed across a wide range of groups and different situations, both academic and physical. Showing someone that a member of a group they identify with has succeeded can make them more likely to succeed, while simply reminding them that they're in a group that tends to do badly at a particular task can make that person do badly. Even something as simple as asking people to tick a box indicating their gender before they take a maths exam can impair girls' performances because of the stereotype that that group is not as good at maths.

'We haven't found anyone that we can't screw up by suggesting that some group they're a member of is bad at something,' said Beilock. Incredibly, as she found in one study, white men will jump significantly lower after you tell them the jumping test is a measure of 'natural athletic ability'.

This has myriad applications across sport: think of Manchester United's knack for scoring late winners under Alex Ferguson, England players' repeated failures to win penalty shoot-outs at international level but not club level, or British tennis players' collective failures at Grand Slam tournaments over the years before Andy Murray. All are examples of situations where a history of group success or failure made subsequent occurrences more likely.

Managers and coaches could tap into this by making sure they steer clear of referring to negative group characteristics and focus only on the positives. As we've seen in this chapter, there are a number of innovative ways to avoid choking, including squeezing a ball in your left hand or humming to yourself. But, when it comes to an English player taking a penalty in a crucial World Cup knockout game, maybe it's best if they think of their club and not their country.

In *White Men Can't Jump*, Hoyle is teased by Wesley Snipes' character for his inability to dunk a basketball, and even though he insists he can, he fails to do so three times when there's money on the line – a classic example of choking. He also claims that when he is 'in the zone', nothing can distract him. The zone is a real place, and the next chapter is about how athletes get there, what their brains look like when they do, and how sports psychologists and scientists are helping them ward off the choke and get into 'flow'.

Try this at home:

PERFORM UNDER PRESSURE

Take down the hijacker

There's nothing you can do to prevent an amygdala hijack. If your brain perceives a threat, it will bypass your conscious mind and send out the hormones that trigger the flight, fight or freeze response. Your heart will race, the blood will rush to your head. What you can do, though, is reinterpret the physiological symptoms when they arrive. Your conscious mind can take what you're feeling and turn it into something constructive, in the same way that the All Blacks use the haka to convert any pre-match tension into an intimidating but controlled display of force.

Get your head out of the game

One of the simplest fixes for paralysis by analysis is to simply give your interfering left hemisphere something else to do. Something as simple as clenching your left hand could help you maintain your sporting performance under pressure. Other athletes have used focus cues – saying a word out loud as they hit the ball in golf or tennis, or singing to themselves to keep the brain busy. Rory McIlroy found that his putting improved when he sped up on the greens. By giving himself less time to think, he stopped himself from overthinking putts.

Train under pressure

The goal when training should be to ensure that your brain has seen it all before, and knows what to do no matter what scenario comes up. This is less practical to implement for the amateur athlete, but you could still work it into your practices: simulate the pressure of a game by making sure something is riding on the outcome, whether it's money, pride or simply the threat of having to run a lap around the field.

CHAPTER EIGHT

IN THE ZONE WITH LEWIS HAMILTON

Lewis Hamilton is flying. Right foot hard on the floor, flicking through the gears, his Mercedes clips the kerbs of the famous Eau Rouge corner perfectly and flies up the hill as the track weaves through Belgian forest. It's August 2015, and the double F1 champion is about to set his 10th pole position of the season at Spa, one of the fastest circuits on the calendar.

I catch up with him a couple of days later at Mercedes-Benz World in Surrey – a glass and chrome construction that's part theme park, part car dealership. He's in a good mood, having won the race to extend his lead in the 2015 F1 drivers' championship, which he'll go on to win. In between talking about his tattoos, his title ambitions and his background in racing, I'm keen to get a sense of how it feels inside his head when everything is going right, like it did in that qualifying lap at Spa.

'I don't really know how to describe the feeling,' he tells me. 'It's all positive. It's just positive energy. You plan for things to happen and when they happen the way you planned them to, it's a good feeling.'

It's a common phenomenon across sports and active pursuits.

Football legend Pele remembers 'a strange calmness' during one of his best performances. 'I felt I could run all day without tiring, that I could almost pass through them [his opponents] physically. I felt I could not be hurt. It was a very strange feeling and one I had not felt before. Perhaps it was merely confidence, but I have felt confident many times without that strange feeling of invincibility.'

'You're ahead of yourself really,' says former F1 driver Mark Webber. 'You really are in slow motion. It's almost being played out before you get there. It is just the ultimate feeling and the ultimate balance of you having the car on the limit, and you're at one, basically. The grandstands could be empty, they could be full – that is not important. You're just completely in a trance of having that car on a tightrope.'

I like these two complementary quotes, one from Ayrton Senna and another about him, showing what this feeling looks like from the outside and how it feels to the athlete. This is experienced F1 driver John Watson talking about what it was like to watch Senna in full flow, in Maurice Hamilton's book *McLaren*: 'I witnessed visibly and audibly something I had not seen anyone do before in a racing car. It was as if he had four hands and four legs. He was braking, changing down, steering, pumping the throttle and the car appeared to be on that knife edge of being in control and being out of control.

'The car was pitched in with an arrogance that made my eyes open wider. Then – hard on the throttle and the thing was driving through the corner. I mean, it was a master controlling a machine. I had never seen a turbo car driven like that. The ability of the brain to separate each component and put them back together with that rhythm and co-ordination – for me it was a remarkable experience; it was a privilege to see.'

And here's Senna himself, talking about the unique sensation of control he felt at times. 'I felt as though I was driving in a tunnel,' he said. 'The whole circuit became a tunnel . . . I had reached such a high level of concentration that it was as if the car and I had become one. Together we were at the maximum. I was giving the car everything – and vice versa.'

This feeling has many names. Psychologists have called it 'peak performance'. Athletes might call it 'being in the zone'. Mihaly Csikszentmihalyi calls it 'flow', and in this chapter we'll explore its incredible power.

The Pursuit of Happiness

Rijeka, a town on Croatia's Adriatic coast, has also had many names and has changed hands many times. When Csikszentmihalyi was born in 1934, it was part of an Italy on the cusp of conflict. As it did for many, the Second World War caused upheaval for the son of a Hungarian diplomat – one brother was killed, another exiled, and Csikszentmihalyi ended up in an Italian prison camp at the age of seven. 'I realised how few of the grown-ups that I knew were able to withstand the tragedies that were visited on them,' he remembered, speaking about his formative years in a TED talk. 'How few of them could even resemble a contented, satisfied, happy life once their job, their home, their security was destroyed. So I became interested in understanding what contributed to a life worth living.'

After attending a talk by influential psychologist Carl Jung (completely by chance because he didn't have enough money to go to the movies), Csikszentmihalyi emigrated to the United States at the age of 22, intent on studying the key components of happiness and answering the question: What makes life worth living?

To find out, he equipped a group of teenagers with beepers that would sound at random intervals during the day. Whenever a beep went off, they had to record their thoughts and feelings. He found that they were unhappy a lot of the time, as teenagers are, but that they tended to be happiest when they were focused on a challenging task. 'The best moments usually occur when a person's body or mind is stretched to its limits in a voluntary effort to accomplish something difficult and worthwhile,' he wrote. He called this phenomenon 'flow', and it shows up in all areas of life, including sport.

Flow has been reported by runners, musicians, surgeons and video-game players – an ancient Chinese text even describes the feeling in a skilled butcher carving up an ox. According to Csikszentmihalyi, who outlined the characteristics of flow, the state can be defined as 'being so involved in an activity that nothing else seems to matter. The ego falls away. Time flies. Every action, movement and thought follows inevitably from the previous one, like playing jazz. Your whole being is involved, and you're using your skills to the utmost.'

If you're like me, and 48 per cent of other people, you might experience flow while doing knowledge work. My favourite and most productive spells of writing come when I'm totally absorbed in what I'm doing. At times like that, the words stream on to the screen in front of me as quickly as I can think. This doesn't happen for everything I write; a lot of the time it's a frustratingly slow experience. But most substantial passages will be cracked in one prolonged burst of activity, a period of intense concentration during which the passage of time seems to speed up. If nothing distracts me, it can be hours before I look away from my screen or pause to do something else. A distorted sense of time is just one sign of flow. Other signs include a loss of the feeling of self-consciousness and a lack of awareness of bodily needs.

Flow is powerful. It can save lives, and it allows people to push the human body beyond the limits of what we thought was possible. In *Bone Games*, author and journalist Rob Schultheis describes it as an almost mystical experience, one he encountered while climbing Mount Neva in Colorado. 'The person I became on Neva was the best possible version of myself, the person I should have been throughout my life. No regrets, no hesitation; there were no false moves left in me. I really believe I could have hit a mosquito in the eye with a pine needle at thirty paces; I couldn't miss because there was no such thing as a miss.'

People are better when they're in flow. They seem to have more time. They make better decisions, and they make them faster. A study by management consultants McKinsey found that top executives in flow are 500 per cent more productive.

Flow can boost creativity for days. Outdoor retail company Patagonia, whose corporate headquarters are on the California coast, have a policy whereby employees are allowed to drop whatever they're doing to go surfing if the conditions are right. The idea is that if they get into a flow state in the water, that productivity and creativity boost will carry over into their work.

In chapter three we looked at some morally dubious techniques such as electrically stimulating the basal ganglia or injecting the brain growth factor BDNF, which could massively increase the level of neural plasticity in the brain, potentially speeding up skill development and breaking the 10,000-hour rule. Flow can do the same. Powerful experiences enhance learning, and flow is about as powerful an experience as you can get. Athletes in flow take in more data and process it more efficiently. Training in flow could 'significantly shorten the learning curve towards expertise', according to performance psychologist Michael Gervais.

Full flow is elusive in traditional sports. When it happens, it's a special, few-times-in-a-career type thing. But it shows up all the time in adventure sports. Surfers, BASE jumpers, even kayakers report the strange sense of power you get when one false move could see you plummeting to your death. They need flow. 'You're immortal, when everything clicks and you're feeling it,' says mountaineer Kenton Cool, who experienced the sensation when he was part of the first team to tackle three of the Himalayas' highest peaks (Nuptse, Everest and Lhotse) in a single expedition. 'Maybe the stars align or the planets align and it's your day, and everything you touch turns to gold. It's a great feeling – if only you could bottle it and bring it out when you need it.'

Flow happens when you're totally absorbed and concentrated on a task with clear goals, which you have personal control over, which offers a good balance between your challenge and skill levels, and which also offers direct and immediate feedback. It could be driving an F1 car, skiing down a particularly tricky slope, writing a book, or even trying to crack a challenging level on your favourite video game. There are thought to be 17 triggers for flow in all, and each of them can be manipulated to enhance or prolong a flow state. The more triggers you hit, the deeper the state of flow.

We've become quite bad at hitting these triggers in certain environments. Take 'focused attention' for example, a prerequisite for flow. As modern technology has made it easier than ever to multitask, we've forfeited some of the ability to lose ourselves in a task for hours at a time. Looking at my desk at the moment, I've got my laptop open, plus a smartphone, a Kindle and a couple of reference books all full of distractions. I have 32 tabs open in my web browser – I just counted them – and going through them is like a geologist digging through various strata of rock. I can see where I got distracted and by what. There's a tab open on a two-hour broadcast of a *StarCraft* tournament (see below), of which I watched the first 30 seconds before opening a new tab to look up what time the nearest supermarket closes. There are several random BBC articles from today's most-read stories column, and the Wikipedia article for the deer tick (which spreads Lyme disease – see below). Needless to say, this is not a productive way to work if you want to get into flow.

Once you're knocked out of the zone, it can take 15 minutes to get back there, if you manage it at all. Open-plan offices are another disaster area if you want to create flow; they're full of constant interruptions, from ringing phones to colleagues coming over to chat.

Athletes do find it a bit easier to focus their attention than office workers, particularly if they're engaged in a dangerous activity. Two other important flow triggers – clear goals and immediate feedback – are also easier to hit in sport than in other settings. A snowboarder attempting something daring has a very clear goal and immediate feedback from their movements as to whether that goal is likely to be reached.

Another key prerequisite for flow is the challenge/skills ratio. The sweet spot is thought to be 4 per cent – that is, the challenge should be 4 per cent harder than your current skill level – difficult enough to keep you interested and improving, but also within reach so you don't lose motivation, and don't hurt yourself trying something beyond your capabilities. Flow is more than automaticity. It only happens when you push at the boundaries of your ability; a difficult challenge, but one that you can raise your game to meet.

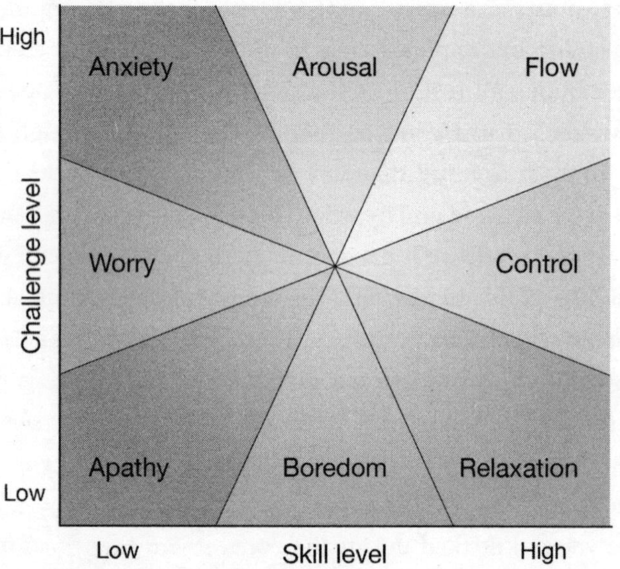

The context also matters. For a full-flow state, it has to matter – something needs to be on the line, whether it's an athlete's life, their livelihood or simply their pride. They need to be in a rich, unpredictable environment where they don't know what's going to happen next, so they're operating at the edge of their abilities. This leads to heightened attention; the brain's processing system kicks up a gear, and you get deep embodiment – a kind of hypersensitivity to the world around that is one of the hallmarks of flow.

I'll Be Back, Dude

Jake Marshall has been wired up like the Terminator. On an overcast day in Salina Cruz on Mexico's Pacific coast, he is waiting for the right moment to strike. The 17-year-old is slight and skinny, with long hair bleached blond by the sun. He is going to be a surfing sensation. He already looks the part and will soon be one of the sport's biggest stars. Right now, though, he's nervous.

He has a laptop strapped to his back, like a London commuter, and he's wearing a specially modified EEG headset, with a swimming cap over it to stop it from getting wet. He also has goggles, and all manner of motion trackers and monitors on various parts of his body. The wires run down from his head into the laptop, where Red Bull's team of researchers back on the beach hope it will be able to record his brain waves as he's making decisions. When he spots a wave he likes and plans to ride, Marshall has to blink three times to create an easily identifiable mark on the recording.

It's the first time a recording like this has ever been done, and the results are revealing. 'There's a rhythm called alpha rhythm, which relates to how relaxed you are,' says David Putrino, the neuroscientist running the experiment. 'In Jake, he's got these amazing bursts of alpha – he's a really chill individual. He's sitting there watching waves, and we're just seeing these alpha waves take control of the recording.'

The waves of the brain's ocean are created by the electrical activity of millions of neurons firing. This is what an EEG measures. They can be broken down into five major types depending on their speed, with each related to a different level of consciousness. Watching the data spool out of someone wearing an EEG cap is fascinating: the lines write themselves on the screen like a seismograph or a stock ticker, some in short jerky movements, others with longer, smoother rises and falls.

Delta, the slowest brain wave, happens when you're in a deep sleep; no dreaming, straight out like a light. Theta is a slightly higher frequency wave – it peaks more often – which is correlated with meditation, REM (rapid eye movement) sleep, and processing new incoming stimuli.

During alpha, everything quietens down, like a calm sea. Beta waves are associated with anything from learning and concentration at lower frequencies to stress and fear at higher levels. Above that, there are gamma waves, which occur in spikes when the brain combines different thoughts into one idea. Flow has been linked to a pattern of alpha waves at 10Hz – waves that peak 10 times a second, which is relatively slow in neural terms.

The patterns of alpha wave activity observed in Marshall's brain while surfing are similar to those discovered by Bradley Hatfield and others at the University of Maryland, who compared expert athletes and non-athletes using EEG. One study of novice and expert shooters also found that the experts' brains showed a drop in neural activity just as they were about to pull the trigger. Their brains showed a decrease in coherence – the different regions of the brain stopped communicating with each other as much as they had been before. Another study of karate and fencing athletes found that their brains tended to run in neutral, that same, quiet, restful state.

The opposite pattern occurs when athletes choke – they can't keep out unhelpful thoughts from the rest of the brain. One study of darts players showed an *increase* in brain coherence when people were watching them, as well as a rise in anxiety levels and a fall in the accuracy of their throws.

This all tallies with what we have learnt about automaticity and choking in the last few chapters. When you're paying attention to a skill, because you're a beginner or because you're under pressure, you think about it consciously and a wide range of brain areas are active.

The better you get at something, the more automatic it becomes, and the less other areas of your brain need to chip in. 'Think of a factory,' says Dr Leslie Sherlin in *The Rise of Superman,* Steven Kotler's book about flow. 'If all the workers are broken into little pods and they're all doing unique things at unique times, that's the explicit system. On an EEG it shows up as beta. Replace those pods with a giant assembly line, one where the work is extremely rhythmic, fluid and collaborative – aimed at a collective goal – that's the implicit system. It's usually denoted by a low alpha/high theta wave.'

God in The Machine

Have you heard the one where seven Tibetan Buddhists and some nuns walk into a psychology department? In 2001, neuroscientists Andrew Newberg and Eugene d'Aquili scanned the brains of the Buddhists and nuns while they meditated. Experienced meditators often describe feeling at one with the universe – similar to how Mark Webber describes being at one with his car in flow.

In this unusual religious gathering, Newberg and his colleagues observed a fall in activity in part of the brain's parietal lobe during meditation, specifically in an area called the orientation association area (OAA). The OAA helps your brain keep track of your body's exact location in space. It is in charge of working out where you end and the rest of the world begins.

When people meditate they deny this area sensory input, so it has no information to work with when trying to draw the borders between an individual and their environment. It is therefore forced to conclude that the individual and the world are one and the same.

A similar thing is thought to happen in flow, but instead of the OAA being deprived of sensory input, it is starved of neural resources. Flow is all about heightened awareness and increased attention, but that comes at a cost. Energy (in the form of blood flow and glucose) is diverted towards those tasks and away from other cognitive functions. This phenomenon is called 'transient hypofrontality'.

In flow, some areas of the brain, particularly in the prefrontal cortex, effectively start switching off. This gives athletes the range of unusual sensations they experience when they're in the zone, including a loss of the sense of self, as the OAA and other areas start to dial down their activity.

'Our nervous system is incapable of processing more than about 110 bits of information per second,' said Csikszentmihalyi in his TED talk. 'And in order to hear me and understand what I'm saying, you need to process about 60 bits per second. That's why you can't understand more than two people talking to you.'

He goes on to use the example of a composer who feels as if his hands are moving of their own accord when he's absorbed in working on a composition – when he's in flow. 'When you are really involved in this completely engaging process of creating something new, as this man is, he doesn't have enough attention left over to monitor how his body feels, or his problems at home. He can't feel even that he's hungry or tired. His body disappears, his identity disappears from his consciousness, because he doesn't have enough attention, like none of us do, to really do well something that requires a lot of concentration, and at the same time to feel that he exists. So existence is temporarily suspended.'

Time slows down or speeds up. Athletes in flow seem to have all the time in the world. This is called time dilation, and it's another symptom of transient hypofrontality. Our perception of time is processed by a number of areas of the brain working together, but so many of these areas go offline during flow that our ability to compute time is distorted.

It is also skewed by the heightened awareness we experience. Because we're focusing intently on something specific, the brain stops multitasking and directs more of its resources towards information processing. Because we're taking in more data per second, each moment seems to last longer. It's why Formula 1 drivers can notice banners in the crowd when they're flying past them at 100 miles an hour, why top-class footballers seem to be one step ahead of the play, and one of the reasons why extreme sports athletes can pull off death-defying feats.

Flow switches off your inner voice of doubt. An fMRI study of jazz musicians and freestyle rappers found that an area of the brain involved in impulse control and self-monitoring is deactivated during transient hypofrontality. People in flow make decisions without hesitating or second-guessing themselves.

This is one reason why flow has been linked to increased creativity. Scientists think they've spotted what the 'Eureka!' moment actually looks like on an EEG – a spike of gamma waves 30 milliseconds before a breakthrough moment. Gamma waves occur when different areas of the brain combine, but this spike only happens as part of the pattern produced by brain activity during flow, as Sherlin explains in *The Rise of Superman*. 'This is where athletes in flow have a huge edge,' he says. 'They're holding themselves in the only state that can produce that gamma spike.'

The Flow Cocktail

StarCraft is a real-time strategy game in which players control the military manoeuvres of one of three fictional races, marshalling resources, constructing weapons and barracks, and sending out scouting missions either against the computer or in online multiplayer. It's absolutely huge, particularly in Asia, where tournaments are televised to millions and star players can rake in hundreds of thousands of dollars in prize money.

On Wednesday 3 August 2005, Lee Seung Seop, a South Korean boiler repairman in his late twenties, entered his favourite internet cafe in Taegu, the country's fourth-largest city. It had more in common with a bar than a cafe, though – dimly lit, with a haze of cigarette smoke in the air. Lee loaded up *StarCraft* and started to play.

Video games are very good at producing flow. In fact, they're specifically designed to do so, which is why they're so immersive. Lee didn't stop playing for 50 hours. When he didn't come home on Friday, his mother asked his former colleagues (he had been fired for showing up to work late after gaming sessions) to go and find him. They tracked him down, and Lee told them he would finish one last game and then return home, but he never made it. 'He just fell off his chair,' said one witness. 'His eyes were closed, he was conscious, but we could tell right away that it was serious.' His cause of death was heart failure caused by extreme exhaustion and dehydration.

This is the dark side of flow. It's addictive. Scientists call it 'autotelic', which means that it's an end in and of itself. It's like a drug. In fact, it's like five drugs – cocaine, speed, cannabis, heroin and Prozac all rolled into one. Flow unleashes the full power of the brain's chemistry, the heady cocktail of neurotransmitters and endorphins that tweak and modify all the electrical activity going on in your head by changing how neurons communicate.

The zone is not a binary state; you can't flick it on and off like a light switch, unfortunately. Not yet, anyway. To get into flow, you have to move through a four-stage cycle, each with its own mix of neurotransmitters that influence motivation, creativity and learning.

The first stage is the struggle phase. It is preparation, and it's generally not that enjoyable. For Lewis Hamilton or Mark Webber, it could be the anxiety and pressure in the run-up to a big race. During this phase, stress hormones like cortisol, adrenaline and norepinephrine are released to boost focus and alertness, and raise heart rate, just as in the fight, flight, freeze response. As well as that, there's a release of the neurotransmitter dopamine.

Dopamine is hugely important in the brain – it underpins our reward system. It's what video game developers target with their games; they're constantly tweaking things to take advantage of this facet of biochemistry, whether it's by rewarding you with coins or points that you can collect and spend in game, or simply by having flashy and stimulating animations when you succeed at something in the game. It's all primed to exploit your dopamine system. When we succeed at something, our brains release a tiny squirt of dopamine, and it feels good.

Dopamine is also released when we encounter something new. It enhances the brain's performance, and in flow, along with norepinephrine, it has an effect similar to the drug speed. It boosts the brain's ability to recognise patterns. People feel like their senses are heightened. They can keep distractions at bay more easily and stay focused on the task at hand.

In the next stage of flow cycle, the release phase, people then have to move all that extra information they're getting from their heightened senses out of their conscious awareness and into automatic processing. That means taking their mind off the problem. Athletes have different ways of preparing themselves: some will spend time with their friends and families until the last possible moment, others will shun all that and seek isolation and peace.

At the end of the release phase, there's a body-wide release of nitric oxide – a signalling molecule that rids your body of stress hormones like norepinephrine, and replaces them with calming neurotransmitters and endorphins to signal the start of flow.

Endorphins are the brain's natural opiates, except a hundred times more powerful. They create the tranquil feeling of being in flow, while anandamide, another neurotransmitter released during flow, works like cannabis – it lifts mood, improves lateral thinking and inhibits our ability to feel fear. Finally, serotonin is also released; this is the neurotransmitter which the antidepressant Prozac acts on. It creates the happy afterglow that athletes feel when they've been in flow.

In athletes, this cocktail of chemicals works together to create that almost invincible feeling of being in the zone. Awareness and focus are heightened, because of the existing rush of 'fight or flight' neurotransmitters and because the brain is diverting resources away from higher cognitive functions to help boost the senses.

At the same time, other neurotransmitters create a sense of calm; there's none of the panic normally associated with stress hormones.

Finally, transient hypofrontality created by the fight for neural resources means that the sense of self is eroded, time falls away, and all that's left is the athlete, their sport, and a feeling of pure enjoyment and skill.

Working together, these neurotransmitters heighten our focus, ramp up our pattern-recognition abilities and improve our lateral thinking, as well as priming our bodies for action. But at the same time they keep us calm, which gives athletes the ability to coolly react to setbacks and make creative life or death decisions in fractions of a second. This is the chemical essence of flow.

We're only beginning to tap into its, and our, full potential.

Mir Cat

Flow changed Steven Kotler's life. 'I got very sick when I was 30 years old,' the best-selling author tells me from his office in Arizona. 'I spent about three years in bed with Lyme disease, and at the end of it there was nothing the doctors could really do for me. They pulled me off medicine. Nobody knew if I was ever going to get any better. I was kind of functional about 10 per cent of the time. I could write and was clear-headed for maybe, like, half an hour a day, and the rest of the time I just lay on the couch, numb. I could barely walk, my mental function was totally gone. No short-term memory, no long-term memory.'

With things looking bleak, a friend managed to drag Kotler to the beach to go surfing. He had been an accomplished adventure sports journalist before his illness, often accompanying the professionals on skiing and surfing trips. 'She kind of had to walk me out to the break, she put me on a surfboard, and muscle memory took over. I paddled a couple of times, and hopped up into this wave, and I popped up into a dimension that I didn't even know existed,' he says. 'My senses were incredibly heightened; I felt like I had panoramic vision, time had slowed to an absolute crawl. I felt better than I had felt in years, and I got better.'

As a sceptical, rational, scientific man, Kotler was thrown by this almost mystical transformation, and he wanted to find out more. 'I was pretty certain that the only reason I was having these quasi-mystical experiences was that the disease had gotten into my brain,' he says. 'The only time Lyme is fatal is when it gets into your brain. I was certain that even though I was feeling better I was losing my mind and it was a symptom that I was dying. So I led out on a giant quest to figure out what was going on, and I quickly discovered that these strange states were called flow states, and there were scientific reasons why I was feeling better. The same neurochemicals that show up in flow all boost the immune system, and they reset the nervous system – they calm it back down to zero. I discovered that this same state of consciousness that was helping me go from sub-par back to normal was helping normal people go all the way up to Superman.'

Kotler went on to write his book, *The Rise of Superman*, on the science of flow, and alongside collaborator Jamie Wheal he co-founded the Flow Genome Project, an initiative aimed at helping people get into flow states and make the most of their transformative powers. 'Every gold medal or world championship that has ever been won, either solo or in a team, we now believe there's a flow state at its heart,' Kotler says. He is a peak performance evangelist who wants to 'hack' flow, and he's not alone.

In the 1960s, the Apollo space programme, America's frantic race to the moon, ran into a problem. Their astronauts were experiencing epileptic seizures and hallucinations brought on by the fumes from their rockets' fuel. At the same time, at UCLA, researcher Barry Sterman was running experiments with cats – a variant on Pavlov's famous conditioning experiments with salivating dogs. Sterman connected his cats up to an EEG to measure their brain waves during the experiment.

A cat would be placed into a room with a lever and an empty bowl, and every time the cat pressed the lever the bowl would be filled with a mixture of milk and chicken broth. The cats quickly learnt to press the lever when they wanted food, so Sterman added a layer of complexity to the experiment. This time, a tone played and if the cat pressed the lever while the sound was playing, they wouldn't get the food. They had to learn to wait until the tone stopped, and then press the lever. Eventually, while waiting for the tone to stop, the cats would remain still and alert, ready to pounce. The EEG revealed something fascinating: a unique, rhythmic pattern of brain waves which Sterman called the sensorimotor rhythm (SMR).

By making the delivery of the food contingent on the brain wave patterns measured by the EEG, Sterman found he was able to train the cats to be able to produce that brain frequency at will – if they produced half a second of it, they got their food.

At this point, completely by coincidence, NASA got in touch with Sterman to ask him to run some tests on monomethylhydrazine, the rocket fuel that had been causing its astronauts and workers such problems. Sterman agreed to test the fuel on his cats, and he found that exposing them to it did indeed induce seizures, as expected. But not in all of the cats. Ten were unaffected – the same ten that had been involved in the earlier experiment on brain waves. Learning to control their brain waves had somehow made the cats resistant to the rocket fuel-induced seizures.

Sterman had inadvertently stumbled on a technique that is now called neurofeedback – the idea that we can improve the brain's performance by training ourselves to get into a particular mental state on demand. The idea quickly caught the attention of the mind-expanding culture of the 1960s and 1970s, which has tarnished its reputation somewhat in serious scientific circles. However, those in the industry now claim that the science has caught up with the technology, and the technique is being used to help stressed-out businesspeople and children on the autistic spectrum, as well as athletes. Chelsea and Real Madrid are among the football clubs reportedly using neurofeedback, while it's particularly popular in individual sports, especially golf.

Brainworks is one company offering sessions in the modern form of neurofeedback, and in their plush clinic near Holborn, in central

London, I get a chance to try it for myself. Clinical director Christina Lavelle hooks me up with the tools of her trade: an EEG cap with 16 electrodes, plus a syringe for squirting in the gel that will connect them to the scalp so my brain waves can be read by her computer. I sit back in a comfortable chair and watch the wall-mounted flat-screen monitor in front of me as Lavelle clicks a few buttons to get things started.

Fittingly, she selects a space-themed game to show me the ropes. Three spaceships appear, each racing along parallel to each other. My brain waves control the speed of the middle one, and the aim is to get it in front. When I produce the right pattern of brain waves, the speed increases, but when I fall out of the groove, the spaceship slows to a crawl and the other two zoom ahead. 'The aim is to not try and do it,' Lavelle tells me. 'Just relax. The more you think about going in front the more you're getting in the way of the brain.'

While I play, Lavelle watches my brain activity live on two screens, and changes settings on her computer, tweaking the weight with which the different brain waves are reflected in the game to make it challenging but not too challenging, and trying to make sure she elicits the desired pattern of thought. In my case, we've decided to focus on concentration, but patients come in with emotional issues, anxiety about performing under pressure, or stress. 'Men like it because they don't have to talk about anything,' she jokes.

The second game I play is more serene. A grassy meadow appears on screen, or, at least, a computer-generated version of a grassy meadow. A scattering of butterflies float around, and my goal is to get them to the bottom of the screen, near the grass. The longer I do this, the more flowers start to appear among the blades of green, and at the same time I rack up points, as displayed in the bottom right-hand corner of the screen.

Treatment starts with an EEG and a questionnaire in which the prospective patient can highlight any problems they're experiencing, as well as lifestyle considerations which could be having an impact on their brain. The number of sessions required can vary wildly, from 10 or 20 to over 100 in some cases, and it doesn't come cheap – a standard session starts at £135. The aim is to get the brain 'in balance', says Lavelle, to improve performance but also to reduce issues with anxiety and performing under pressure. As well as the EEG, Lavelle's range of tools includes a brain stimulation kit and 'Heart Math' – a heart-rate monitor which can be used for 'biofeedback', a similar process whereby people learn to bring their heart rate under control.

Neurofeedback practitioners want to train the brain to produce a particular pattern of brain activity, but not just in the session itself; they want to get those changes to stick, by altering the neural pathways the brain uses. 'The reason we usually say 20 sessions is because we want it to move and we want it to be permanent,' says Lavelle. 'We reinforce that a number of times to override the old patterns. The reason it stays permanent is because it's a nicer, more comfortable and pleasant way to be.'

Some of this sounds a bit New Age, a bit pseudoscientific. In the 1960s and 1970s. neurofeedback devices were featured in mail order advertisements in the back of magazines such as *Yoga Journal*, and scepticism lingers. Indeed, the jury is out on whether neurofeedback has any scientifically verifiable, tangible benefit beyond what would be offered by a placebo. But athletes seem to like it, and Lavelle defends her work. 'The reason neurofeedback is getting more and more popular is because it works,' she says. 'We're getting more and more busy because of word of mouth and that's because it works. I get people coming in and after one session they notice the difference.'

New technology (or newly packaged old technology) means that you don't necessarily have to go into a clinic to train your brain. The Versus headset arrives in a slick black package. It consists of a pair of over-ear headphones of the kind you might wear in a music studio, right down to the garish black and fluorescent yellow colour scheme. But in this case the headband portion forms a cross over the top of the head. At the points and at the centre of the cross are small, inch-square grids of half-inch-long black, rubbery protrusions, like the bristles of a hairbrush. These are the electrodes in this do-it-yourself neurofeedback kit – one group at the front, one in the middle, one at the back and one on each side. I connect the headset to my iPad with a headphone cable, and then press a button on the side to switch on Bluetooth and connect it with that as well.

In an 'on-boarding' session over Skype, a San Francisco-based customer service rep talks me through the process of putting the headset on. First, take the sensor conditioner, which comes in a small pot and looks like lip balm, and apply it to the electrodes. This is the slightly less messy version of the conductive gel used in a traditional EEG. Then position the headset on your head, wiggle it back and forth and pull it down firmly to ensure a good connection to the scalp. The app features a top-down illustration of a head which glows green to indicate the strength of the connection, and can show you your brain waves in real time.

After that, I complete an assessment of my brain activity, which mainly involves sitting still with my eyes closed while the headset and app record what's going on in my head. Once that's done, it recommends a training programme on some of the app's many training games: NeuroShapes, NeuroBalloon, NeuroGlider and NeuroRacer are some of the ones I try. They're fairly similar to the games I tried in a more formal setting at Brainworks – the speed and movement of my avatar depends on my brain activity, whether it's a racing car, a hot-air balloon or a wingsuit pilot. Some of the games incorporate a degree of movement as well; I can tilt the iPad left or right to navigate through rings in NeuroGlider, for example. This can have the effect of helping you take your mind off your own brain activity, letting the brain get into a relaxed state by itself. At Brainworks, Lavelle shows me a similar programme which changes the brightness of a video being played – the better the brain activity, the brighter and easier to watch it gets. 'You might feel like you forget what you're doing,' she says. 'This is great for kids as well because we can put cartoons on.'

SenseLabs, the creators of the $400 Versus headset, recommend using it three times a week for eight weeks to see tangible results. It's proving popular among athletes already, including tennis doubles legend Mike Bryan, who has won 16 Grand Slam doubles titles alongside his twin brother Bob.

'I think everyone plays their best tennis when they are relaxed but their mind is turned on,' says Bryan in an interview with *tennishead* magazine. 'I have been using the race car, which only moves if you are in the optimal brain state. They don't give you any instructions, you just look at the screen and the car will only move if you are in the zone. Your brain figures it out. It's crazy – all of a sudden the car will jump forward a little bit. Then the car starts moving so your brain figures out where it needs to be. You can feel the blood flowing to your head which is kinda cool. It's like working a muscle. You can feel yourself getting really tired after 20 minutes.'

Dr Leslie Sherlin, one of the founders of SenseLabs, claims that using the headset has helped get Bryan out of unhelpful patterns of anxious behaviour he would become trapped in after losing points, and helped him recuperate mentally after matches. 'Mike has what we call a very high neurostrength,' Sherlin has said. 'He is really good at being able to engage at a really high level, but his weakness is around the ability to turn that off, either in between sets or between matches. Being able to fully reduce the cortical activity enables maximum recovery.'

Bryan claims the headset has helped his game. 'I've noticed my tennis has improved,' he continued. 'I can concentrate longer. Our matches are generally an hour-and-a-half and before my concentration would waver during that time but now it is easier to sustain that focus, which is huge. Sleep has been a big difference too. Sometimes I'm a restless sleeper but I've been sleeping better. And I notice during the day I'm not as irritable and my memory seems a little better, too. When I'm really stressed I'll just throw on the headset and it'll bring me back, bring my breathing down and get me back in a good rhythm.'

Debbie Crews has a more tangible measure of the improvement that neurofeedback can provide in a sporting context. She's been working with another at-home neurofeedback headset called the Muse headband, which looks like something a *Star Trek* character might wear to communicate with the *Enterprise* while on a hostile planet. As well as linking up to a visual display of brain activity, the Muse's accompanying app also uses music as feedback, which Crews is using to train athletes through her recently founded company Opti International.

'We like to use music because then they can be up in their putting stance or hitting a ball,' she says. 'What happens is, they've got the headset on and they're going to go through their routine, and the music is going to be going up and down. But just before they release the pitch or just before they start the club back the music needs to be low, and that's going to be representative of synergy in the brain. Their brainwaves are running the music, and if you do it repeatedly it's really neat because they learn to lower their music and it becomes really consistent over time.' She's seen results. 'I did a study last summer, and we improved putting performance over and above physical practice by about 16 per cent.'

Neurofeedback is also helping people to get into flow states. Chris Berka is now CEO of Advanced Brain Monitoring, a company that makes high-end EEG headsets for use in research (they're the ones Sherwin and Muraskin have been taking to baseball teams). But before that, she conducted a fascinating bit of research using neurofeedback. She found that when she trained novice marksmen to control their breathing and manipulate their brain waves on a screen in front of them, they were able to produce the alpha waves found in flow at will. The time it took them to learn how to shoot like professionals fell by more than half. 'So Malcolm Gladwell's famous 10,000 hours to mastery,' says Kotler, 'what the research shows is that flow cuts it in half.'

All that these high-tech solutions and headsets are doing is training and helping people to control their thoughts. Of course, you don't need expensive equipment to do that, as the Buddhist monks and nuns prove – they too produce the alpha activity found in flow. 'Mindfulness meditation is another way to do this,' says Kotler. 'All these neurofeedback devices, all they're doing is training focus in the same way as any mindfulness meditation practice.'

At the Flow Genome Project, Kotler and team have developed their own mindfulness training programme centred around a video called *The Art of Flow*. I ask him for one tip people can implement themselves. 'The easiest answer is the simplest answer,' he says. 'Regulate your breathing. It sounds so stupid, but if you're breathing really shallow, fast, anxious breaths you're producing too much cortisol, stressing your body out too much, and it's going to block flow.'

Identical twins Steve and Nick Tidball have developed a unique way to try to encourage this behaviour. In the 1980s, a series of experiments found that a shade of pink called Baker Miller Pink could suppress aggressive behaviour in prisoners. The pair worked as creatives in the sports industry before starting their own company, Vollebak, to pursue their goals in another arena – endurance racing. The Baker Miller Pink hoodie is designed to be worn in the moments leading up to a race, to calm nerves and encourage a flow state. As well as the unique shade, it features a mesh screen which zips up over the wearer's head to encourage slow, controlled breathing.

Equipment and clothing design have already been used to shave seconds off in the swimming pool and on the racetrack, but combining this with what we know about the brain is a newly developing field, and one that could help athletes get into a state of flow. It's far from the only method being tried, though.

Just Beet It

According to the label, Beet It organic beetroot juice has a natural, earthy taste. I think it tastes like soil. I'm sipping it, rather tentatively, because according to Kotler drinking beet juice is a potential shortcut to flow. This better be worth it.

This particular brand is cut with apple juice to, and I quote, 'smooth out' the earthy tones – but you can buy concentrated shots of the stuff in specialist sports shops to dilute with water, or, if you're particularly sadistic, mix in with your porridge of a morning. Beetroot juice also turns your urine pink, as I was slightly alarmed to discover a few hours later.

Athletes drink it because it's packed with nitrates, which are already well known to aid endurance by boosting blood flow to the muscles and making the conversion of food into energy in the cells more efficient. During London 2012 some teams struggled to find beet juice because so many athletes were buying it. It may also help to get you into flow by providing your body with the resources it needs for the release of nitric oxide, one of the neurochemical precursors to a flow state.

This surprisingly thick purple liquid is just one of the ways Kotler and others are trying to hack flow, although they're yet to see 'any results worth a damn' from beetroot juice – something I contemplate as I admit defeat and tip the rest of the bottle down the sink.

Flow hacking, as Kotler calls it, involves practising with different flow triggers. Throughout his book, Kotler uses case studies of extreme sports athletes – skateboarder Danny Way, BASE jumper Dean Potter, kayakers and snowboarders. His rationale is that the progress extreme sports athletes have made over the last few decades is utterly remarkable, and it's all down to flow; their sports are rare in that they have all the ingredients required. To help those of us less inclined to leap off cliffs take advantage, he's designed what he calls a 'flow dojo' – a kind of adventure playground for adults.

Inside, there will be trapezes, human gyroscopes and all manner of contraptions designed to give your body the sensation of risk, but in a safe environment. When I speak to Kotler, the project is deciding between two competing sites – one in Utah and one in Colorado – for their 'extreme playground equipment'.

It's not just a playground, of course; there's a bit of science going on as well. Participants are wired up to all manner of headsets to measure their heart rate, the g-forces they're being exposed to and, of course, their brain activity (by means of the same Versus headset used for neurofeedback). By training people to take the adrenaline rush of movement and turn it into alpha waves in their brain, the flow dojo can help them open the door to a flow state and all the benefits that brings.

One of those benefits is a rapidly increased rate of learning. A 2011 study by DARPA, the US military's advanced research division, found that snipers trained in flow were 2.3 times quicker at finding their targets. Training in flow cut the time it took amateur snipers to shoot like experts by 50 per cent. 'Flow can radically and rapidly change the brain permanently,' says Kotler. 'Think about the neurochemicals in flow – they're all rooted in the basal ganglia.'

The basal ganglia is a deep and vital part of the brain's primitive machinery. In chapter three we saw how neuroscientists have been experimenting with reopening critical periods for heightened neural plasticity by electrically stimulating the basal ganglia. Flow might be able to do the same thing, only naturally.

The Resurrection of The Dallas Cowboys

The Super Bowl of January 1993 ushered in a new era for the NFL's showcase event – an era of big-name stars being asked to play the half-time show. They kicked it off with a bang. Michael Jackson seemed to appear on top of the giant video screen in a corner of the Rose Bowl in Pasadena. A couple of seconds later, he leapt on stage in the centre of the field, launching into a medley of his greatest hits once the screams from the crowd had subsided.

Meanwhile, on the sidelines, something much more interesting was going on. The Dallas Cowboys were on the rise; they were being rebuilt under new coach Jimmy Johnson, who had taken over a few years previously. Now, with his side 28-10 up at half-time in the Super Bowl, an interviewer asked him what he had changed to help prepare his side for the biggest game of their lives. He held up a copy of Csikszentmihalyi's book, *Flow*, and explained that the team had used it as an integral part of their preparation in the days leading up to the game.

Flow is not just confined to individuals. Its most powerful applications may well be when people work together in harmony – group flow. The Cowboys forced a record nine turnovers of possession in that game, three of them leading to touchdowns in the first half. They were playing, collectively, on a different level.

Professor Keith Sawyer is one of the leading thinkers in the field of group flow. Approaching it from a musical standpoint, he wanted to get an idea of what was going on when an orchestra or a jazz band clicked together to create something truly special. 'At any second during a performance, an almost invisible musical exchange could take the piece in a new direction; later, no one could remember who was responsible for what. In jazz, the group has the ideas, not the individual musicians,' he writes in *Group Genius*. It's like a school of fish suddenly changing direction all at once.

Group flow is powerful stuff. One study by psychologist Charles Walker compared solitary flow, co-active flow (where athletes share an environment but don't co-operate) and interactive flow (where interaction is key to success), and found that participants experienced higher 'flow enjoyment' when their activity was more social. Another study of more than 300 employees at a strategy consulting firm which Sawyer cites in his book found that the highest performers were those who participated in group flow.

This is clearly highly applicable to sport. Group flow helped the Dallas Cowboys win back-to-back Super Bowls in the early 1990s, and there's surely an element of it in the way that top football teams like Bayern Munich or Barcelona pass and move together. They say certain midfielders can pass the ball 'with information on it', and in football group flow is what is happening when everyone knows what their teammates are going to do. 'The best players are the quickest thinkers,' said Barcelona midfielder Andres Iniesta in an interview with *FourFourTwo*. 'Where is my teammate going to run to? Will he stay onside? Which one has space? Which one is looking for the ball? How do they like the ball – to their feet or in front? You can be the best passer in the world, but without your teammates being in the right position, it's no good.'

A number of the 17 flow triggers relate specifically to group flow. One of them – blending egos – is perhaps the most interesting one for sport. Blending egos means that everyone needs to contribute; the team can't be geared towards one or two stars. It could explain why players sometimes struggle when they move clubs.

A company called SyncStrength is using heart-rate data to try to measure team chemistry. The theory is that the more in sync players' heart rates are, the more likely they are to perform better together. This effect has been found off the field: married couples whose heart rates are more in sync have longer, more stable relationships, for example. At the Sloan Sports Analytics Conference in 2013, Dan McCaffrey and Kevin Bickart, the founders of SyncStrength, presented two examples from football of players' heart-rate synchrony. In one, players' heart rates seemed to align when they scored a late winning goal; while in the other, the team conceded, and the player who had lost the attacker she was supposed to be marking was out of sync with the rest of the team. A confirmed link between heart-rate synchrony and performance could give coaches a quantifiable way of measuring whether their team is clicking, whether they're in group flow.

'Group flow gives us the outer extreme of co-operative possibility,' Kotler tells me. 'It's the state of ultimate co-operation. The idea that you and I can get in a flow state together and feel like one organism – that idea was total nonsense, laughing-stock-lock-you-up-in-a-padded-cell nonsense, 20 years ago. We've gone from that to this idea of a co-operative hive-mind. We have no idea what the upper limits are and that's what I think is so interesting. We're much better at working with individual flow than we are with group flow, and we don't even know what the upper limits of individual flow are yet. We think we've tapped about 10 per cent of our actual potential. It's hugely exciting.'

In Part Two, we've looked at how neuroscience is helping athletes train better, perform under pressure and get into the incredible state called flow. In Part Three, we'll look at how neuroscience is revolutionising sport in other areas. It's helping us understand the pressures sport can put on the brain and how to manage them, whether it's contending with a lack of oxygen at high altitude or the trauma of concussion. It's also shedding light on what makes athletes in dangerous sports seek out risk, and aiding scouts in their search for the great sporting brains of the future. But we'll start with endurance – another area where unlocking the secrets of the brain could help push the limits of human performance.

Try this at home:

SHORTCUTS TO PEAK PERFORMANCE

Listen to your brain

Neurofeedback devices such as the Versus headset are helping people control their brain activity and produce the same pattern of alpha waves found during flow. Learning to control your brain activity through neurofeedback could help train the brain to produce the pattern of activity found during flow in a sporting context, and build neural pathways that will make it easier to get into the zone when you're playing.

Control your breathing

You don't have to splash out on expensive neurofeedback sessions or a do-it-at-home kit, or choke down earthy beetroot juice. Buddhist monks and nuns in meditation show a similar pattern of brain activity to people in flow, and you can unlock some of the benefits of flow, such as a release of relaxing endorphins, through meditation. But the easiest way to improve your chances of getting into flow is to simply control your breathing. By doing so, you'll help release the calming endorphins and neurotransmitters that, when combined with those released during the flight, fight or freeze response, trigger a hyper-productive flow state. 'If you're breathing really shallow, fast, anxious breaths you're producing too much cortisol, stressing your body out too much and it's going to block flow,' says Kotler.

Pull the right triggers

Flow happens when you're pushing at the edge of your abilities, so whatever activity you favour, make sure you're not stuck in a rut. Get out of your comfort zone and challenge your skill level, but don't go too far. The sweet spot is thought to be around 4 per cent – the challenge should be 4 per cent harder than your current skill level to maximise flow. You can maximise the chances of flow in other areas of your life by eliminating distractions. Turn off alerts on your phone or from your email account, minimise any background noise, and you'll find it much easier to get into hyper-productive flow state.

Part Three

THE NEXT SPORTING REVOLUTION

CHAPTER NINE

RUNNING THROUGH THE WALL

Robbie Britton is not in a good state. He sways like a drunk, eyes unfocused and staring blankly into the middle distance, dark hair matted down with sweat. One of his support team looks concerned. 'Just keep moving forward,' the ultra-marathon runner is told as he stumbles on, pausing only to rinse his mouth with water from a plastic bottle, and then spit it out on to the tarmac. It's 23 hours into the 24-Hour World Championships, a competition that pushes the human body to the limits by challenging athletes to see how far they can run in a day.

'It's a 24-hour race done in a loop,' explains Britton when I speak to him on the phone – he's in the Alps training for the Ultra-Trail du Mont-Blanc, another gruelling endurance race. I've just asked him to tell me the worst state he's been in during a race, and he directs me to a YouTube video depicting the scene above. 'In the video I've just thrown up two litres of Coca Cola, and I stumble in to see my crew and they're talking to me,' he says. 'I just look like I'm drunk, like a complete mess.'

The brain suffers as much as the body in situations where we're pushed to the limits. Endurance racing's triple whammy of sleep deprivation, boredom and the sheer mental willpower required to keep moving forward can lead to some interesting sights. 'I've seen some weird shit,' says Britton, as he tells me about a 153-mile race in Greece where he ended up falling asleep on a garden wall in the middle of the course. 'I remember looking forward, looking for my crew. There was a little field to the side and I remember seeing a load of meerkats in there. It's kind of dawn, early light, and when I look up close I realise it's not meerkats, it's deer. You see what you want to see, and apparently at that time I wanted to see meerkats, because that would have cheered me up no end! People say they hallucinate – at times your eyes play tricks on you in the early hours of the morning.' That is a problem sometimes compounded by the strange get-up favoured by spectators of distance races. 'I remember seeing a guy at the end of the race: a six-foot-four bloke in a silver suit, with a silver cane and top hat,' says Britton. 'And he was actually there!'

Kilian Jornet, another ultra-runner and one of the world's best (he ran up and down the Matterhorn in less than three hours), has had auditory hallucinations. 'You hear people or helicopters or animals, and you're in the wilderness so there's nobody there. I have friends that say they've seen the trees attack them, or they've seen a bed and they just want to sleep in the bed and then they fall, because obviously it's not a bed . . .'

Physical fatigue affects mental decision-making across all sports. One study of experienced orienteers found that it greatly impaired their ability to process visual information. Cricketers bowl less accurately when they're dehydrated. Tennis players' ground strokes are almost 70 per cent less accurate after 35 to 40 minutes of exercise.

Britton recalls one extreme example of faulty decision-making induced by fatigue and dehydration. 'I've overtaken someone who was running the wrong way up the course. I had to correct him and tell him to turn around – he didn't believe me. He was fucked; he hadn't drunk properly and then he decided that running the opposite direction to which he was supposed to go was the right thing to do.'

Often, especially at the very top, success in sport comes down to who can make the right choice in a crucial moment, who can win the final point of an epic five-set tennis match, or pick the right pass with aching legs in the last moments of extra time in the World Cup final. Athletes are generally better than amateurs at maintaining their mental performance under physical stress. In this chapter, we'll discover how our new knowledge of the brain is helping them get even better, and how training your brain could help you push yourself further and faster.

Return to Base

There's a BASE jumper throwing up in the bathroom. I'm back at the Human Performance Lab, observing an experiment being conducted by Dunlop Tyres to test how some of their athlete ambassadors respond mentally when put under physical pressure. Under supervision by Professor Vincent Walsh of University College London, a group of five athletes from varied sports are going head-to-head with average members of the public (in this case, a group of magazine journalists).

First, they head to the lab's computer testing room to establish a baseline level of mental performance. They complete a reaction-time task in which they have to quickly identify shapes and patterns. Then they take on the Iowa Gambling Task, a test of their ability to assess risk and probability.

After these tests, the participants are taken into the HPL's main area, where two exercise bikes have been set up side by side. To a soundtrack of frantic shouted encouragement from Walsh and his team of assistants, they push themselves to the limit for two minutes, in 30-second bursts of maximum effort. It's a really difficult thing to do. By the end, everyone is sweating, gasping for air, no matter how conditioned they are. Unfortunately for them, it's straight back into the computer room for a repeat of the psychological tests.

Winter Olympian Amy Williams, who won gold in the skeleton for

Great Britain in 2010, is one of the athletes participating, and I spoke to her afterwards as she refuelled in the HPL's equivalent of a green room. 'After the bike test I was really dizzy,' she says. 'I couldn't see properly, I was really wobbling. My legs were jelly. We went into the computer test room and it hurt just to sit down – my legs, the lactic acid. I was really fidgety; I was trying to stand up, shake my legs out. I was resting my head on my arm and just really struggling.' BASE jumper and wingsuit pilot Alexander Polli put so much effort into the task that he had to make an unscheduled bathroom visit to, for want of a more delicate phrase, puke his guts out.

Still, despite the clear physical stress they were under, this informal test confirmed that elite athletes had the edge when it came to maintaining their mental faculties. Take the visual search task, for example, where both elite athletes and non-athletes had to identify objects on a computer screen. Initially, there wasn't much difference between the groups – both took around 630 milliseconds per object on average. When they took the tests again after their bike tests, a vast difference emerged. The non-athletes' performance deteriorated significantly, as you might expect. They took 932 milliseconds on average to find each item – 82 per cent worse than the elite athletes.

The athletes actually *improved* under physical pressure; they were more than 100 milliseconds quicker per item on average. Their performance in the Iowa Gambling Task also improved three times more than the non-athletes the second time around.

One reason could be that athletes are better at blocking out any physical pain or fatigue they might have been feeling. 'I knew I had to finish the task,' said Polli when I spoke to him after he'd recovered from his efforts. 'The headache and the nausea were coming on quite strong, but I can't say I was really too affected because it was kind of like I didn't even have a choice. I didn't have a choice to give the headache attention or to give the nausea my attention – somehow I was able to zone them out.' Williams felt the same. 'You were very aware of telling yourself to concentrate even though you know you were tired, you still sort of self-talked yourself. You were still very much, "No, come on, you've got to do this."'

Another thing that set the athletes apart was their level of commitment to the physical task itself. They were much more inclined to push themselves to near their true limits, revealing a real difference in mentality, even in a situation with nothing riding on it except pride. 'Half of us athletes were the ones who were almost throwing up in the toilets, passing out,' says Williams. 'I really, genuinely, couldn't have given any more – but could the non-athletes? Actually they probably could have done another set, and that's the thing, isn't it? I don't know whether I could have done another set. I would have, because I would have been told to. You kind of think, "Well, I'm not gonna stop until the person says stop"; you just do it, and you give it all and you keep going. Whereas someone else might be like, "Well, I'm getting tired, so I'll back off a bit."'

The Longest Day

John Isner knows all about not giving up. The American tennis player was the winner of the longest match in his sport's history at Wimbledon in 2010, finally prevailing over Nicolas Mahut after 11 hours and five minutes of play spread over three days. He won 70-68 in the fifth and final set. Isner said that the mental fatigue was as hard as the physical during the ordeal, and that's actually true of any sport that requires athletes to push their physical limits. The very act of forcing yourself to keep running around the court or keep going in an endurance race requires effort from your brain.

'We shouldn't underestimate how much mental effort an endurance race requires,' says Professor Samuele Marcora, one of the world's leading experts on the subject. He is based at the University of Kent, where he has conducted a range of studies with athletes looking at how the brain deals with fatigue. Marcora hails from Italy, and though he admits that he's not much of an athlete himself, he claims endurance experience because of his love of motorbikes. He once rode all the way from London to Beijing, going through Tibet's high mountain passes en route. When I speak to him, he's just back from a working trip through four European countries, all done on the back of a motorbike. With that recent experience perhaps still running through his mind, Marcora explains that ignoring the signals coming from aching feet or groaning muscles is hard work, mentally.

'You start to have pain, or get tired, or sleepy – all of your body is telling you to stop. Especially in those ultra races, it's not really natural; it's not something that the body is especially happy to do. So it's going to send you a signal in terms of pain, in terms of tiredness to stop or to slow down considerably. In order to perform, you need to inhibit this natural response, and response inhibition is a very demanding cognitive activity.'

Willpower actually requires mental power, in other words, and exercising that mental power can be detrimental to your physical performance.

Marcora has tested this using an experiment called the Stroop test, which you may have come across before. It involves reading out a list of names and colours, which are printed in different-coloured ink, creating a mismatch. So the word 'black' might be printed in yellow ink, for example. Participants are usually asked to read the ink colours out loud, while resisting the temptation to say the word. It can be surprisingly difficult, and is a classic test of response inhibition – the same skill required to ignore the signals telling you to stop running or cycling.

There have been a number of studies along these lines, but one fairly typical example was published in 2014. Two groups of participants were asked to do a Stroop test. One group had the ink colours and words matched, while in the other they were mismatched to tax the brain's powers of response inhibition. Immediately afterwards, both groups were asked to run 5 kilometres on a treadmill. On average, it took the group who had done the response inhibition task more than a minute longer to cover the distance.

Monotonous mental tasks can have the same effect because you have to exercise willpower to keep concentration. In another experiment, one group of cyclists was asked to do a letter-recognition task for an hour and a half, while another group watched a documentary about the Orient Express train. Then, they were asked to cycle as hard as possible for as long as they could. Those who had watched the documentary lasted 12.6 minutes on average, while those who had been doing the monotonous letter-recognition task lasted just 10.7.

When findings like this first emerged, they shattered the accepted view of fatigue. 'If you look at the two tasks you think, "Well, why should playing in front of a computer for 90 minutes affect high-intensity exercise?"' says Marcora. 'That's something which in our field has always been thought to be limited by your cardiovascular system or the energy content in your muscles.'

Fatigue doesn't just come from the body. It comes from the brain.

Grinding up Frogs

The annals of neuroscience and medical research are full of gruesome experiments that wouldn't look out of place in a horror movie. One of the most important studies in the field of exercise physiology, conducted in 1907 by Nobel Laureate Sir Frederick Gowland Hopkins, fits that description. The paper describes a method for grinding up the limbs of frogs in a mixture of ice and alcohol in order to measure the lactic acid contents of the muscles (or create the worst cocktail imaginable). This study was one of the first to demonstrate that lactic acid builds up in muscles in the absence of oxygen – it's what gives you that burning feeling in your arms and legs during strenuous exercise, as your lungs can't take in enough oxygen to feed the muscles.

This finding set the field on a track that persisted for almost a century. It led to a view of the heart and lungs as the limiting factor in exercise. It was thought that as long as the muscles had oxygen and energy available, they would keep contracting until they ran out of energy or too much lactic acid had built up. Our bodies were thought to be like cars – you could drive until the petrol ran dry or something in the engine broke.

The notion of a 'brainless' exercise physiology persisted largely until the 1990s, when South African physician Dr Tim Noakes revived a forgotten idea that has become known as the 'central governor' hypothesis. It suggests that the limiting factor preventing you or me from running for as long as Robbie Britton or Kilian Jornet is not our bodies at all, but our brains.

If you ask people to exercise until they can't go on any longer and then analyse their muscles by biopsy, as one study published in *The Journal of Physiology* did, you discover that biologically speaking their muscles could have kept going at the same rate for another seven or eight minutes. People give up long before they reach their metabolic or muscular limit.

You can see this in the way endurance athletes are able to rapidly increase their pace towards the end of a race, a so-called 'end spurt', when their brain realises that there's not much more exertion left. 'I did the 24-hour World Championships again in April and my fastest 10 kilometres of the race was my last hour. I was running under three-hour marathon pace,' says Britton. 'In reality, my body should have been in bits, but I knew I had a chance of an individual medal.' Their muscles should be exhausted, according to the old theory, but they're able to keep going and squeeze out a little bit more effort because the brain relaxes its tight control when the end is in sight.

It's not a conscious process. The central governor is thought to operate along the lines of other biological processes such as temperature control. The body is designed to maintain a state of homeostasis – stability. So when you eat sugar, for example, the pancreas will release insulin to bring your blood glucose levels back down to normal. When you're hot, the blood vessels near the skin will automatically dilate to release some of that heat.

'The central governor hypothesis suggests that within your brain there is a controlling mechanism which unconsciously prevents you from over-exerting, from running or exercising beyond certain limits, and controls the pace you would have in a race to keep it in safe limits,' says Dr Thomas Rowland, author of *The Athlete's Clock*. 'This governor is a beneficial governor because it prevents you from injuring yourself. There are very real possibilities with over-exertion that you can break bones, shred muscles, have a lack of coronary blood flow to the heart muscle. All these things could happen, but they don't and that's the evidence that there's some controlling mechanism, out of our control, that says you're only going to go this fast.'

It fits in with what we know about other mechanisms that maintain our body's stability. It has evolved to prevent itself from self-destructing, and so according to the central governor it would not make sense that you could injure yourself by overexercising.

However, overprotective brains can be the biggest barrier for athletes in pursuit of records. After Roger Bannister broke the four-minute mile, a host of others soon followed his lead, suggesting it was more a psychological barrier than a physical one. The two-hour marathon is arguably the equivalent in this era, and our brains are one factor as to why it hasn't happened yet. 'When you start running,' says Noakes, in Ed Caesar's *Two Hours*, a book about the quest to break that milestone, 'you know what the world record is, so you don't have to run ten minutes faster than the world record. Your whole focus is to run one second faster than the world record. That's what your brain is keyed in on. And that programming occurs all the time in running and is terribly important.'

Finnish runner Paavo Nurmi, who won nine gold and three silver medals in the Olympics for distance running, seemed to know this already. 'Mind is everything,' he said, in a quote that Noakes uses in one of his papers. 'Muscles are pieces of rubber. All that I am, I am because of my mind.'

One Man March

According to some estimates, there were a million people locked outside the Olympic Stadium in White City, London, on 24 July 1908. They had come to see the climax of the marathon, which finished, as is now traditional at the Games, with a lap of the athletics track. A marathon is 26 miles and 385 yards exactly. It takes its name from the Battle of Marathon in ancient Greece in 490 BC, when Pheidippides, a messenger, supposedly ran from the battlefield to Athens to deliver the message that the Persians had been defeated. According to legend, he ran the entire distance without stopping, delivered his news, and then collapsed and died – an early blow for the central governor hypothesis.

The route between Marathon and Athens is approximately 26 miles, and the modern-day marathon is based on that distance, although not exactly. The extra 385 yards owe their existence to Princess Mary of Wales. In 1908, the race was due to start outside her residence, Windsor Castle. However, the starting point was moved inside the grounds so that the princess's children could watch, which accounts for the extra distance still added to marathons today.

The additional yards would prove crucial, particularly for Italian runner Dorando Pietri, who took the lead in the race with two miles to go. Sir Arthur Conan Doyle was one of the lucky 100,000 crammed into the stadium, and what happened next was as gripping and dramatic as any Sherlock Holmes story.

The 22-year-old Pietri entered the stadium to a roar from the crowd, but unfortunately the trained pastry chef could not translate that support into a powerful finish. He fell several times in the final 400 metres, and had to be helped up by the race umpires, which meant he was disqualified after the race had ended.

'As I entered the stadium the pain in my legs and in my lungs became impossible to bear,' wrote Pietri in an Italian magazine seven years later. 'It felt like a giant hand was gripping my throat, tighter and tighter. Willpower was irrelevant now. If I hadn't been so bad I would not have fallen the first time. I got up automatically and launched myself a few more paces forwards. I no longer knew if I was heading towards my goal or away from it. They tell me that I fell another five or six times and that I looked like a man suffering from paralysis, stumbling with tiny steps towards his wheelchair. I don't remember anything else. My memory stops at the final fall.'

The point is that this doesn't sound like a man whose brain is protecting his body, so perhaps the central governor, although it's a neat concept, is not quite the correct one. That's what Marcora thinks; he prefers what he calls the 'psychobiological model of endurance'.

According to his way of thinking, there is no central governor, no area of the brain that receives signals from the body and tries to maintain a state of homeostasis. He still believes that our endurance is limited by the brain, but more simply by our motivation and our own perception of the effort we're exerting. 'It's pretty clear that highly motivated people in certain situations can push themselves to a point where the body's homeostatic control cannot cope,' he tells me. 'For example there are cases, famous pictures of heat stroke and triathletes wobbling to the finish line, which partly demonstrate that there's no central governor because otherwise they wouldn't be able to push themselves to death.'

So, according to Marcora, it's not about how much work our muscles have actually done, but how much our brains think they've done. 'If I block all the signals from your legs at a spinal level with anaesthesia – an epidural – your perception of effort doesn't go down to zero,' he says. 'People always take for granted that perception of effort originates from sensory signals from the body, from muscle, temperature, oxygen receptors sending signals to the brain. But it doesn't. Perception of effort doesn't come from the body – it comes from the brain itself.'

Instead of your brain receiving feedback from the muscles, in this model it's the intensity of the neural signal being sent out that determines how the brain perceives the effort being exerted. It's like working out the speed of a car not by measuring it directly or looking at the speedometer, but by looking at how hard the driver is pressing his foot down on the accelerator.

Muscles are bundles of fibres which contract or expand depending on the movement and force required. The more powerful the movement, the more muscle fibres you have to contract, so the stronger the signal your brain has to send down to them. As you exercise, some of these fibres get tired. Fatigued muscle is weaker, so in order to run at the same speed or move with the same force as before, you have to recruit more muscle fibres because each one is pulling less powerfully. The brain has to send out a stronger signal to recruit those extra fibres, and this is how it measures perception of effort.

What this all means in practice is that if we can control our perception of effort, we can take the handbrake off and push our bodies beyond what we thought was possible.

After his defeat to John Isner in that monster tennis match, Nicolas Mahut had something of a breakdown. Following a special on-court ceremony to mark the longest match in the sport's history, and the awarding of commemorative champagne flutes to two players who clearly just needed to lie down (this is very Wimbledon), he had to be carried the last few metres back to the locker room by his coach, as reported by Ed Caesar in *GQ*. He wept, and found it hard to stand or breathe. He couldn't remember anything about the closing moments of the match. 'Did I lose the match, or did he win it?' he kept asking his coach, who had to carry him into the shower, fully clothed.

Incredibly, he was back out on the same court three hours later playing in a doubles match, while Isner was interviewed on the terrace above. A week later, he sent Isner an email underlining what he'd learnt from that gruelling encounter. 'Everything that had been written about my physical and mental boundaries was wrong.'

Silencing Demons

Simon Wheatcroft is planning to run across the Sahara desert. Looking at his running CV, there's no reason why he shouldn't be able to do it. He has completed the London marathon, the 100-mile South Downs Way race, and he once ran all the way from Boston to New York, staying at strangers' houses on the way. He is also almost completely blind. Wheatcroft started losing his sight at the age of 17 due to a degenerative condition called retinitis pigmentosa, but he hasn't let it limit his ambition.

In his late twenties, he started running alone on a loop near his house, using only the changing conditions underfoot and the RunKeeper iPhone app to help guide his way. On new routes, he runs with a guide, but for training he has honed his technique and memorises how sections of road feel so he knows what is coming up.

He puts his determination down to one incident. 'I went to climb a mountain over in California, the Half Dome,' he tells me. The Half Dome is one of Yosemite National Park's most famous structures – a granite peak rising almost a mile. 'The idea was to climb to the top and propose to my girlfriend and to make it this incredible moment. I'd never climbed a mountain before, but I figured it wasn't going to be that hard. It turns out it is quite hard.'

Ultimately, Wheatcroft was forced to abandon the attempt on grounds of safety, but vowed never again to let his visual impairment, or anything else, stop him from completing a task he'd set himself. 'I told myself from that point that I'd never quit again – no matter how hard physically or mentally it becomes, quitting is no longer an option,' he says. 'So I began this journey to chase down the point where it becomes difficult just to see if I could stand back up.'

That's what led him to his first 100-mile race in the Cotswolds, a huge leap into the unknown in many ways. Wheatcroft had never run that far before.

Fifty miles in and he was slumped, head in hands, in a support vehicle. 'The reason I was so destroyed was that I learnt to train solo outdoors at an airport, which is pancake flat for a good reason, and the course that I'd picked was incredibly hilly. Because I'd done all the training alone I'd never actually run up a hill because there were just no hills to run up. I ran 50 miles of severely undulating route and the pain was just becoming difficult to manage – my legs were really sore, I was starting to blister really badly on my feet. I got to that 50-mile point and I broke down. I burst into tears; physically I was just destroyed. I didn't even know if I could carry on any further, but I thought to myself, "I can't quit – it's not an option."

'I couldn't quit, but I *could* accept failure, and the only way you're going to fail is if you can no longer stand. So I told myself I would keep going until I could no longer stand. I got out of the van and ran for 33 more miles until that point did come where my legs just gave way. I had someone either side of me holding me up, and I couldn't actually move my legs no matter how much thought I put into it.'

Wheatcroft's story proves that the mental wall can be scaled, and scientists all over the world are finding ways of making it easier by studying what happens in the brain when people push themselves to their limits. Dr Kai Lutz, a neuropsychologist at the University of Zurich, has used EEG caps to measure the brains of cyclists and find out what happens when they give up. He found an increase in communication between the motor cortex, involved in the planning and control of movement, and the insular cortex, which processes signals from elsewhere in the body, at the point of failure. Lutz suggests that the insular cortex is where distress signals from the body are monitored; that it is the part of the brain with its foot hovering over the brake, if you believe the central governor hypothesis.

One of the problems with investigating the brain during endurance exercise is that it's quite difficult to do any kind of exercise within the narrow confines of an fMRI machine. But a team of researchers in Brazil have developed an ingenious contraption which allows a participant inside a scanner to cycle while lying on their back, with a series of gears and cranks connecting their efforts to a fixed exercise bike. Using this machine, they scanned the brains of seven people while they cycled on and off for 15 minutes, and asked them to also rate their perception of effort at intervals during the test. They found activity in an area of the brain called the cingulate cortex, which tallies with Marcora's work – this area of the brain seems to be involved in calculating the perception of effort. It's the same area that is involved in weighing up the merits of potential choices during decision-making.

A lot of what we know, or think we know, about the human brain comes from animal studies – damage a part of the brain and see what the subjects, in this case rats, can and can't do. In one study, which Marcora told me about when I asked him which areas of the brain were implicated in the perception of effort, rats were faced with a T-maze. To the left, a small amount of cheese; to the right, a larger amount of cheese. The catch, in this plentiful world of cheese, is that the larger haul is behind a barrier and the rats have to exert more effort to climb over and reach it.

Normal rats will do the extra work to get the extra cheese, but rats with a damaged anterior cingulate cortex won't. They'll take the easier option for the smaller reward, even though they can still sense that the larger reward is simply a climb away. 'The experiment shows very dramatically that this area is associated with effort, and decisions based on effort,' says Marcora.

Whether you subscribe to the central governor model, or believe it's our perception of effort that limits us, it's becoming clear that our heads quit before our bodies. Yet our muscles have incredible, untapped strength. In a TED talk, journalist David Epstein uses the example of the way people are flung across the room when they get electric shocks – that's the full power of all our muscle fibres contracting at once.

The limiting factor in endurance is not our muscles or our lung capacity. The limiting factor is the brain, but it can be overcome. 'Our brain acts as a limiter, preventing us from accessing all of our physical resources, because we might hurt ourselves, tearing tendons or ligaments,' explains Epstein. 'But the more we learn about how that limiter functions, the more we learn how we can push it back just a bit; in some cases, by convincing the brain that the body won't be in mortal danger by pushing harder.'

A Shot in The Arm

Tom Simpson's final words were widely misreported. News travelled slower in those days and, on the way down from the punishing slopes of Mont Ventoux, the words were twisted and turned, until they reached a journalist in a bar down in the valley, who embellished them further for the back pages of the *Sun*.

Ventoux looks like it's snow-capped all year round, but when you get closer you realise its upper slopes are totally barren. The winds that give the mountain its name scour it of plant life. That leaves no shade for weary riders in the Tour de France, on one of the race's toughest climbs – a steep vertical ascent of almost a mile.

The climb was even tougher on the summer's day in 1967 when Simpson made his last ascent. As the peloton inched up the incline on stage 13, the mercury reportedly reached as high as 54°C. The British rider, an Olympic medallist and former world champion, had been suffering with stomach pains and diarrhoea during the crossing of the Alps, and had been unable to eat properly for days. He had been advised to quit the race the night before. He didn't.

On the upper slopes of the mountain, Simpson started to lose control of his bike, zigzagging back and forth across the road. With a kilometre to go to the summit, he fell. 'Put me back on my bike!' are the words commonly attributed to him, but according to his mechanic, Harry Hall, his last words were actually, 'On, on, on.'

And on he went. He climbed on to his bike and managed to ride a short distance before falling again, unconscious, with his hands locked to the handlebars. He was taken by police helicopter to a hospital in nearby Avignon, where he was pronounced dead. How, despite every human instinct, had Simpson managed to override his brain and ride himself to death?

The answer could be found in the rear pocket of his racing jersey: a half-full tube of amphetamines, along with two empty ones, which he had apparently been washing down with brandy during the race. Doping wasn't banned in cycling in those days, and it was endemic. Strychnine and amphetamines were commonly used to dull pain and to aid endurance.

Marcora says that stimulants such as cocaine, or even caffeine, can reduce perception of effort and improve endurance. 'A lot of people originally thought their effect on performance was because they facilitated fat-burning and therefore spared the energy reserve in the muscle,' he says. 'But the reason is they have an effect on your brain. It's the psychobiological effect of these drugs rather than the cardiac or metabolic effects that have an effect on endurance.'

Dopamine has been identified as the key neurotransmitter in perception of effort, and drugs that target the dopamine system already exist. They could also theoretically be used to improve endurance. Some are already on the banned substance list. Marcora does point out, however, that reducing fatigue by medical means is not necessarily a bad thing per se and that working out how to reduce perception of effort in athletes might have wider-reaching benefits. 'Sport is one thing, and a lot of these potential discoveries in terms of doping become illegal in sport,' he tells me. 'But I came from clinical research. If you're a cancer patient and you're knackered after chemotherapy and you can't go to work and maintain your family, your life is really affected. Why not have some drugs that reduce that fatigue and that high perception of effort? It's the same with EPO [erythropoietin, which is used as a performance-enhancing drug in cycling and other sports]. My mum, she was on dialysis for many years and now she has a kidney transplant – she takes EPO all the time. For her it's not doping, it's actually something really good.'

There are less dubious ways to improve your sporting endurance, of course. Good old-fashioned training is one of them. Being physically fitter improves your endurance because it reduces your perception of effort. If your muscle fibres are stronger, fewer of them need to be recruited to do the same amount of work, and so it's less mentally taxing as well. Being in a flow state also improves perception of effort – neurotransmitters are released which deaden pain, and transient hypofrontality (the reduction in activity in the prefrontal cortex) takes you out of your body.

Another common way for athletes, both elite and amateur, to keep themselves going is through self-talk – telling themselves why they have to keep going, or that they just need to make it to the next lamp-post or checkpoint. 'It's not even internal, it's external,' says Britton. 'I'm shouting and talking to myself.'

Some of the work of traditional sports psychologists helps athletes develop and use these mental tools, and they have a proven effect on perception of effort. One study found that using selected self-talk phrases, such as 'drive forward' and 'push through this', could reduce the perception of effort by 50 per cent and increase the distance covered by 18 per cent on average.

There are other ways that athletes can smarten up their training routines. Take John Isner, for example. Why was he able to overcome Mahut? It's partly down to Craig Boynton, his coach at the time, who realised that five-set matches, particularly on grass, can often develop into sprawling affairs settled by a handful of key points. So, as reported by Caesar in *GQ*, he decided to train Isner's 'concentration muscle' – his brain. Isner trained in Florida, much hotter and more humid than London, even on the city's stickiest days. Boynton had him doing three- or four-hour sessions in the heat to build up his endurance and his ability to concentrate while fatigued. 'When they stepped off the plane at Heathrow,' writes Caesar, 'the temperature was in the low twenties, and there was not a cloud in the sky. Boynton turned to Isner and said, "Johnny, look at this weather – you can play ten hours in this."'

Marcora is pioneering what he calls 'brain endurance training' – tasks specifically designed to train your mental endurance (your concentration muscle), so that when your physical limits are tested you'll be able to respond. He has found truly remarkable results. 'You have a physically fatiguing task, which is the exercise,' he explains. 'And on top of that you have this very highly mentally fatiguing cognitive task. You make your training session more demanding to the brain, and if you repeat this over time it will induce other changes in the brain, reduce your perception of effort and increase your performance. That's exactly what happened in our study.'

Working with the Ministry of Defence, Marcora trained two groups of 14 soldiers on fixed exercise bikes over a 12-week period. The two groups saw a similar improvement in their physical fitness, as measured by their VO_2 max – a commonly used indicator of how much oxygen the body is able to get to the muscles. But they varied vastly on a 'time to exhaustion' test, where subjects are asked to ride at a fixed percentage of their maximum possible level until they can't anymore. The control group's time to exhaustion improved by 42 per cent. The group that performed a mentally fatiguing exercise alongside physical training improved 115 per cent.

Mentally fatiguing doesn't necessarily mean difficult. In fact, sometimes, the more boring the task, the better. One task involves looking at an array of arrows on a screen and pressing a button to indicate whether the middle arrow is pointing left or right as quickly as possible. Pretty straightforward, but do it for 90 minutes straight and your mind will feel like it's just run 20 miles.

Doing a boring task releases a substance in the brain called adenosine, which is associated with mental fatigue; it builds up when you're running a marathon, for example, or when you're lacking sleep. One of the reasons coffee is favoured as a liquid wake-up call through much of the world is that caffeine blocks adenosine – which is also why it's been found to improve endurance performance and why athletes often ingest it before races. Marcora has conducted experiments with high-dose caffeine gum, and initial results suggest it can reverse the decline in physical performance caused by a mental task.

Even just training your response inhibition abilities on a computer may improve your physical endurance, according to a preliminary study conducted by Marcora. But he says that doing the mental training while exercising will have the biggest benefit because, as we saw in chapter three, exercise can aid neural plasticity.

Marcora is now working with Axon Sports to develop cognitive tasks for iPhone and iPad that people can do while they're out running. 'At the moment we're using tasks which are visually based so you have things on the screen you have to respond to,' he says. 'We want to develop some auditory response inhibition tasks. People will hear some sounds or the music going off beat and they have to respond, and because they don't have to look at it they can run.'

Until these products hit the market, though, Marcora does have some advice for those of us looking to improve our running endurance. As well as normal training runs, try to schedule some longer-distance, lower-intensity training sessions for when you're more mentally tired – after work rather than before, for instance. 'If you go out for a 20k run after a hard day at work, you'll be experiencing the same level of mental fatigue as you would if you ran 50 or 60km when you're not mentally fatigued.'

After training like this, your brain will be better equipped to cope with the distance; you'll have trained your response inhibition under fatigue, and you'll be less inclined to give up when it counts.

Damn Right, It's Better Than Yours

Indulge yourself with this rich and creamy blend of all of our premium ingredients – sumptuously smooth ice cream, satin whole milk, and sweet vanilla.

Get sensible with the new light healthy Sensi-Shake. It has all the taste, without the guilt – no fat, no added sugar and only 180 calories.

Participants in this study probably couldn't believe their luck when they saw the flyer – getting paid $75 to taste some milkshakes. The 50 people who responded to the ad were given either the indulgent high-calorie milkshake, or the sensible low-calorie option, and before drinking them they had to read a detailed description like the ones above. The researchers measured the level of the stomach hormone ghrelin, which controls how full you feel.

After they drank the indulgent shake, the ghrelin levels in the subjects dropped, just as they would after they ate a big meal. And when they drank the low-calorie shake, their ghrelin levels stayed largely the same as before. So far, so normal. Except that both milkshakes were identical. Simply by changing the label on the milkshake, the researchers were able to completely alter the way the stomach behaved.

The brain, for all its wondrous abilities, is very easy to trick. We see it all the time with the placebo effect – doctors prescribing sugar pills or performing sham surgeries have found real health benefits. Studies have revealed that just rinsing your mouth out with a drink containing carbohydrates can improve your performance and reduce your perception of effort. Sometimes, having less information, or the wrong information, can actually be better, especially when it comes to endurance.

This kind of deception can help people to eke out improvements over and above what they thought were their limits. It's basically what Simon Wheatcroft did in his first 100-mile race – he found the strength to override his brain and get more from his muscles.

Professor Kevin Thompson at Northumbria University asked cyclists on exercise bikes to try to keep up with a computer rider on a screen in front of them until the finishing line. They were told that the virtual rider's speed was determined by one of their own personal bests, so the rider would be travelling at a speed they knew they could manage.

In fact, the virtual rider was going faster than the personal best – up to 5 per cent faster – yet all the cyclists were able to keep up with it, thus improving their own personal bests. 'These findings demonstrate a metabolic reserve exists which, if it can be accessed, can release a performance improvement of between 2 and 5 per cent in terms of their average power output,' said Thompson. 'We believe a small deception of the brain can enhance performance. Despite the internal feedback to the brain being heightened by the extra power output being produced, the participants still believed it was possible to beat their opponent.'

This could be incorporated into training in many ways. Red Bull's performance scientists did something similar for one of their tests in a velodrome. They set up a ring of LED lights around the inside of the track, which the riders then had to chase, like a greyhound chasing a rabbit at the dogs. The riders were told that the light represented their fastest time from the previous day's testing, but it was actually a slightly faster version of themselves. It wouldn't even need to be that complicated – as Mark McClusky points out in *Faster, Higher, Stronger*, something as simple as a fast-running stopwatch could induce you to beat your personal best.

That's not the only way fiddling with the dials can yield an increase in performance. At the Human Performance Lab, there's a chamber with a treadmill in it where researchers can change the temperature and humidity to put athletes through their paces, whether they're triathletes preparing for the Olympics in Rio, or polar explorers looking to acclimatise before they head to the ends of the earth.

Generally, the hotter it is in the chamber, the harder it is for athletes to keep going – hence the opprobrium surrounding the World Cup in Qatar, and why the fastest marathon times are set in places like New York and London. The central governor hypothesis would argue that the body senses the temperature and decreases its effort accordingly. But one study in 2011 found that tinkering with the thermometers so that they showed the wrong temperature could influence performance.

Athletes' performances in the study worsened as you'd expect when the conditions went from normal to hot and humid, but those who were told it was cooler could overcome this effect. They had a lower perception of effort, and they were able to ride harder.

The problem with placebo-style deceptions like these is that if the athlete knows about them, they don't really work. So Marcora and others are working on ways to reduce perception of effort that tap into our subconscious mind.

The light, wraparound sunglasses favoured by some athletes already feature some pretty advanced technology. In future, they could hold the key to endurance-racing success, or find themselves on the banned items list alongside the full-body swimsuits which helped shatter records in the swimming pool. Products such as Google Glass – a heads-up display that is worn as a pair of glasses – can provide information on the go, and a company called Recon make a sturdier version designed for sport. They can flash up information about distance travelled, pace and heart rate like a sports watch, without forcing the runner to take their eyes off what is in front of them.

Marcora has been working with Recon to develop a product that takes advantage of a phenomenon he and his former colleagues at Bangor University in Wales discovered in the lab. They paid 13 volunteers to pedal an exercise bike at a set pace for as long as possible – a common test of physical endurance. But, unbeknown to the cyclists, a screen in front of them was flashing up subliminal messages – for just 16 milliseconds at a time, one-twentieth of a blink. Cyclists who were flashed sad faces rode 22 minutes and 22 seconds on average, but those who were shown happy faces reported less perceived exertion and rode for three minutes longer. 'The brain is very sensitive to faces,' says Marcora when he tells me about this. 'They can really change your brain activity and your mood, so when people are flashed the subliminal happy faces they perceive less effort and they last longer.' Your own facial expression is a good way of measuring perception of effort, so Marcora is also trying to find out whether changing your expression – by smiling while running, for example – can improve your endurance.

He has found the same performance boost with subliminal presentation of words: cyclists flashed action words such as 'Go' or 'Lively' lasted 17 per cent longer than those flashed inaction words such as 'Toil' or 'Sleep'.

You might think that flashing the images up for longer would have more of an effect, but you'd be wrong. 'Some of the stimuli actually work better when they are subliminal than when they are conscious,' says Marcora. 'It's a different kind of brain. They were not conscious of the stimuli, but the unconscious stimuli had a conscious effect because they felt lower perception of effort when they were flashed the faces, even though they didn't see them.'

This is the technology he's hoping to build into the goggles – a subliminal boon for everyone from the amateur runner to the professional that could work to improve endurance, even if you know it's coming.

Brain Zapping

There's something very strange going on in a converted red-brick warehouse in Santa Monica, California. It's a world away from Castle Frankenstein, but inside scientists are pushing the boundaries and harnessing electricity to do things that would have seemed unnatural a few years ago. Tim Johnson is lying back, eyes closed, with a plastic tube emerging from his mouth and wires leading from a plastic cap on his skull to an array of computer monitors. He's covered in sweat, and from time to time his legs twitch powerfully, but involuntarily. To the untrained eye, it looks like he's being tortured.

This is Red Bull Project Endurance, the drinks giant's attempt to help the athletes they sponsor improve their performances, and shift a few more units as well, of course. They've summoned a group of their athletes to headquarters to undergo a punishing series of physical tests, all while they're wired up and analysed in a wide range of ways.

The composition of their breath is being measured, as is the power of their calf muscles and the beating of their hearts. Their brain waves are recorded using EEG caps, and their muscles are induced to twitch using transcranial magnetic stimulation (TMS).

Johnson is a cyclo-cross rider. Cyclo-cross is a physically demanding sport in which riders on lightweight bikes race over wooded trails, or down steep hills over uneven ground. Later, two electrodes are placed on opposite sides of his head, and a current flows between them, changing how likely the neurons in an area of brain are to fire – making it either slightly more likely, or slightly less. This technique is called transcranial direct current stimulation (tDCS). By targeting certain areas of the brain, such as those involved in calculating perception of effort, you can potentially help athletes push through the barriers of endurance.

Mountain biker Rebecca Rusch was one of the athletes to take the test. 'My first thought was, "How is this different from the electroshock therapy they did in the 50s?"' she told Alex Hutchinson in *Outside* magazine. 'I was, like, they're going to do what to my head?' Actually tDCS is a much calmer, almost meditative process – 20 minutes of lying back in a leather chair as the current flowed through her primary motor cortex. 'It feels like very small ants crawling on your scalp,' writes Hutchinson.

There are a number of ways in which brain stimulation could potentially improve performance in sport. 'One is during or just before the performance,' said Nick Davis, a neuroscientist at Bangor University. 'If you're nervous, a little brain stimulation could damp down your muscle responses, a bit like beta-blockers [which are most commonly prescribed to prevent heart attacks]. Another is during training, when it could help you to focus.'

Endurance is another target area. A group of Brazilian researchers gave 10 cyclists 20 minutes of tDCS and found that their power output was improved by 10 per cent. A group of researchers in Italy found that tDCS of the motor cortex improved endurance time for arm movements by more than 15 per cent. It doesn't add extra power to your muscles; it unlocks what is already there. TMS and tDCS have also been linked to shortened reaction times, and improved learning of complex motor skills.

They could, moreover, help people get into a flow state. In the last chapter, I mentioned how a study by DARPA found that training snipers in flow improved how quickly they learnt. But one of the most fascinating things about the study was the way the researchers got their subjects into flow to begin with.

It doesn't take much power – a two-milliamp current will do the trick. With the snipers, Michael Weisend from the Mind Research Network in New Mexico targeted the current through the brain's object-recognition areas, with the aim of making the neurons in the region more responsive.

As well as enhancing object recognition, Weisend found that passing a current through this area led to similar feelings as those observed during flow – calm, focused concentration and improved performance. 'The number one thing I hear people say after tDCS is that time passed unduly fast,' Weisend told *New Scientist*. It's thought this method of stimulation works to induce flow because it reduces brain activity in the prefrontal cortex, artificially inducing the state of transient hypofrontality found in flow.

'tDCS is very easy, and very cheap,' says Marcora. 'You can go on the internet and buy a kit.' Indeed, several companies are already producing tDCS devices purporting to improve focus and mood – you can clip them on to your forehead. There's also a small but dedicated community of people building their own devices at home. All you need is a sponge, some saline solution and a nine-volt battery.

However, there are doubts over the safety of such devices. I wouldn't recommend it. 'Brain stimulation shouldn't be taken lightly,' said Davis. 'As a medical procedure it's fine, but it's not safe to do "in the wild", and there might be long-term effects that we still don't know about.'

Some are sceptical of its efficacy, including Vincent Walsh, who led the fatigue study at the HPL at the start of this chapter. 'Brain stimulation might make you better at something in the lab,' he told the Dana Foundation, 'but that's under conditions where you're pressing buttons in a dark room. You're not under any pressure to win, and you don't have memories of how badly you played in the past five minutes.

'The gains seen in the lab are statistically significant, but they're not necessarily behaviourally meaningful, and there's absolutely no evidence that any of it translates to the real world.' Another point Walsh raises is that these devices are not yet practical enough to be applied in the chaotic world of sport. 'It'll be very difficult to apply it when people are actually doing stuff,' he says, 'and it's pretty unlikely that the effects would have a lasting effect in the rough and tumble of sport.'

I got a sneak peek at what devices designed specifically for sport might look like in the future if they do manage to work out those problems when I paid a visit to The Imagination Factory. Based on an industrial estate in Chiswick in west London, they essentially have the job of thinking big.

Co-founders Julian Swan and Mark Hester threw some ideas at me for where this technology might go in the future, which they're currently taking to sports clubs. Some are more plausible than others. One that caught my eye was a digital design of a helmet with sliding electrodes or TMS coils on it which could be positioned and controlled remotely. 'You could have a coach fiddling with the dials on the touchline to dial up or dial down a player's aggression,' was one of the suggestions.

'It's an interesting potential use of this technology, but it smacks of desperation,' says Walsh, more generally. 'We don't want a generation of kids thinking they need a bit of brain stimulation. It loses the essence of sport.'

It's definitely something the World Anti-Doping Agency might have to look into sooner rather than later. 'Strategies that modulate neuronal activity during training or during sport competition will lead to benefits comparable to those of using drugs,' said Dr Alexandre Okano, one of the tDCS researchers from Brazil, in an interview in the *Globe and Mail*. 'In addition, there is no known way to reliably detect whether or not a person has recently experienced brain stimulation.'

In this chapter, we've seen how the brain controls how far we can push our bodies, and how, by training or tricking the brain, we can overcome those mental barriers. Brain stimulation takes that a step further. It could be the ultimate performance-enhancing drug.

Try this at home:

TAKE THE HANDBRAKE OFF

Tire out your brain

By doing a mentally fatiguing or boring task and then going out to exercise, you're stretching the brain's powers of response inhibition – its ability to ignore the signals from the body telling you to stop. Samuele Marcora suggests mixing up your training routine – scheduling some longer runs for after work will make your brain feel like it's covered extra distance, so when it comes to a race, it will be used to the feeling. It's all about training your 'concentration muscle'.

Knowledge isn't power

In these days of smartwatches and high-tech treadmills, it's easier than ever to know exactly how far you've run, how many calories you've burned, how fast your heart is beating. But it might be better not to know. Giving athletes false information about their performances has been found to reduce perception of effort and increase performance. It's hard to fool yourself, but try switching off the screens – you might find that if your brain doesn't know how hard you're working, it'll let your body push for longer.

Have a coffee

When you're doing a task that requires mental willpower, either because it's boring or exhausting, a substance called adenosine builds up in your brain. It happens pretty much the same whether you're working on a dull spreadsheet or running a marathon, and it contributes to the feeling of mental fatigue you experience. Fortunately, caffeine blocks the effects of adenosine, so having a cup of coffee before you go out for a run could help improve your endurance.

Smile!

Subliminal messaging seems to be another way of reducing your perception of effort. Flashing people smiley faces while they run helps them last longer, and Marcora is working on goggles that can deliver these subliminal messages. He's also exploring the possibility that your own facial expression could impact on your perception of effort. The results aren't in as yet, but running with a smile could be the amateur athlete's secret weapon.

CHAPTER TEN

PASSING OUT IN POLAND

There are a number of warning signs scattered along the 12 miles of tarmac that wind their way to the top of Pikes Peak in Colorado. Mountain lions and black bears are the biggest threat to hikers, but there's even a reportedly serious 'Big Foot Xing' sign, which reads: 'Due to sightings in the area of a creature resembling "Big Foot" this sign has been posted for your safety.'

That's not a concern for Guy Martin, who hopes to be travelling so fast that no sasquatch can keep pace. Martin hails from Lincolnshire, and doesn't look a million miles away from a mythical creature himself, with wolfish unkempt dark hair, wild eyes and a manic grin. He races motorbikes, mostly in insane events like the Isle of Man TT. In 2014, he went to Colorado to attempt the Pikes Peak International Hill Climb, the second oldest motorsport event in America after the Indianapolis 500.

Pikes Peak climbs to more than 14,000 feet, which presents a unique challenge not only to the self-built bike Martin has brought with him, but also to his brain. At altitude, the air is thinner, which means less oxygen for combustion engines and for the brain. An engine runs with 30 per cent less power at altitude, as it needs oxygen to combine with fuel to turn into forward momentum. The brain is the same – its cells need oxygen to fire. Before he went for his attempt on Pikes Peak, which was filmed by Channel 4 as part of a four-part documentary series called *Speed*, Martin went to see Samuele Marcora at his lab at the University of Kent to find out about the effects of hypoxia – a lack of oxygen – on neural function. This chapter looks at the environmental pressures placed on the brain by certain sports, from a shortage of oxygen at high altitudes to the effects of extreme g-forces on racing drivers and aerobatic pilots.

Above around 6,000 feet, the lack of oxygen starts to bite. For travellers, it usually manifests itself as light-headedness, a splitting headache, and an overwhelming desire to stop sightseeing and go and lie face down on a hotel bed. But poor endurance, muscle weakness and impaired brain function are the relevant consequences for sport. To prepare Martin for the challenge to come, Marcora sets him up on an exercise bike inside his own atmospheric chamber, where he can control the oxygen levels. First, though, a 10-minute exercise at sea level, with a test of focus where Martin has to respond to a target appearing on the screen as quickly as possible while riding as hard as he can on the exercise bike. As you might expect for a TT rider, he found it pretty straightforward.

Fast-forward to the next test, and Martin is making the kind of noises you might expect from someone who had actually happened across Big Foot on Pikes Peak. Marcora has dropped the oxygen level from the 21 per cent we're used to breathing in normal air down to 16 per cent to emulate the thinness of atmosphere at the top of the mountain. In the same test as before, Martin is gulping, gasping for air, as Marcora spurs him on with words of encouragement, standing nearby to catch him if he passes out. 'It sounded like a murder scene,' says Martin afterwards, grinning like a maniac. 'I was sort of struggling to see. Maybe 30 seconds or a minute longer and I would have passed out.'

That's not all – his brain speed suffered too, with processing speed falling by 15 per cent. 'You could see his reaction time really plummeting,' Marcora tells me. Not ideal when you're piloting a bike at hundreds of miles an hour.

You'll be spotting a pattern by now. Just like the body, the brain can be trained to cope with the altitude, although, alas, there aren't any clever tricks or iPad apps to help with this just yet. You can train at altitude, as many athletes do anyway, particularly long-distance runners. If you're lucky and have access to an atmospheric chamber, or just have a spare room, lots of plastic sheeting and a hypoxic generator, you can exercise in low oxygen conditions to prepare like Martin did for Pikes Peak.

Or – and this proves there is a technological approach to pretty much every problem nature can throw at us – you can do what Pikes Peak record holder Sebastien Loeb did when he made the ascent in a rally car in just over eight minutes, and get an oxygen mask.

Turbulence Expected

Hanging upside down, high above the Baltic Sea, I can feel my vision starting to fade. Grey circles are appearing at the edges of my sight, so, as I've been instructed, I tense my stomach muscles to try to counteract the g-force pushing the blood out of my head and sending me towards unconsciousness.

I've come to Gdynia, a sprawling port town on Poland's northern coast, for a round of the Red Bull Air Race – an aerobatic flying competition in which pilots navigate their aircraft through a course of inflatable pylons in the quickest time possible. Crowds of locals pack the concrete settlement's pretty beach, soaking up the surprising Polish sunshine and drinking cheap beer as they watch the light aircraft manoeuvre their way around the circuit just metres above the sea. A few miles away, above a military base which is serving as the race airport, I'm trying not to be sick.

I'm in a twin-seater aircraft piloted by Juan Velarde, a stubbly blue-eyed Spaniard who flies in the Challenger Cup, the feeder series for the

Air Race. He has taken me up for a taste of the demands placed on the pilots' bodies and brains by g-force.

G-force will be a familiar phrase for fans of motorsport, but everyone experiences it. It's what pushes you back into your seat when you're in a rapidly accelerating car, or from side to side on a swerving rollercoaster. It gives you that fluttering in your stomach when you go over the crest of a hill on a country road, and the unpleasant jolt of sudden turbulence on a bumpy flight.

When you get into a car and it starts accelerating, your body wants to stay where it is, but the car is moving around it, so as you're being pushed forward by your seat you feel a force in the opposite direction pushing you backwards – that's the g-force. Similarly, if you round a sharp bend, your body wants to keep moving in a straight line, so you feel a push into the side of your seat in the opposite direction to the way the car is turning.

It's not strictly a force, but a way of measuring the effect of acceleration and deceleration relative to the earth's gravity. The force of the earth's mass pulling you down is 1 g. When pilots pull 10 g in a steep turn, this means their body effectively weighs 10 times as much. Trying to move your arms and legs under high-g is like wading through treacle.

We're interested in the brain, though, and as Velarde demonstrates barrel rolls, loop-the-loops and banked turns, I can feel the effects on mine, even though I'm facing a mere 6 g at most, compared to the 10 g the pilots will face on some of the toughest turns on the course. The phenomenon I'm experiencing as my brain drains of blood is known as 'grey-out', as two-time Air Race champion Paul Bonhomme explains. Bonhomme is a neatly groomed 49-year-old Brit who splits his time between flying tiny light aircraft as fast as he can 15 metres above the ground, and piloting 747 jumbo jets for British Airways. I don't know whether to be reassured or concerned.

'We try never to grey-out,' he tells me, as we chat in his team's hangar on the day before the Gdynia race. 'But the way it feels is you feel the g-force coming on and it's like you're being squashed into your seat. The blood pressure is lost from your head, which means the blood pressure in your eye is then lost and you lose vision. So the first thing you might see is spots, or your peripheral vision will diminish and you might have a central tunnel. If you're actually flying yourself, that's the moment where you go "grrrr" and really pressurise yourself to stop any more blood pressure loss in the head.'

He grunts, not unlike the Hulk, and tenses his stomach muscles, which is one of the main ways pilots can counteract the effects, as it slows down the rate at which blood can flow away from the head by squeezing the blood vessels in the torso. It's like closing a lane of traffic on a motorway. Handy tip: you can also do this if you get a head rush from standing up too quickly.

On the other side of the paddock, I meet Bonhomme's Air Race rival Nigel Lamb, who explains more. Lamb is a 57-year-old who lives in Oxfordshire, but his accent marks him out as a former citizen of Africa. He was born in Rhodesia (now Zimbabwe), 'as far away from any flying activity as you could get'. But his father was an aircraft pilot during the Second World War and Lamb caught the flying bug and joined the Rhodesian Air Force at 18, before leaving for the UK in 1980 to become one of the most celebrated aerobatic pilots in the world.

'The most important thing about g-force is you have to relate it to time,' he explains. 'If you jump off a table, you're going to subject your body to quite a lot of g, but only for a nanosecond, so it doesn't really matter. It's all about time, and the ability of your fluids to flow down your body.

'We can easily get to 9 or 10 g in these planes. It's not a problem if it's for a very short period of time. The moment you go into several seconds at 7 or 8 g, you're getting into a territory where you really have to pay a lot of attention because of what's called G-LOC.'

G-LOC stands for 'g-force induced loss of consciousness'. 'The greying of your vision is quite a nice warning signal,' says Lamb. 'If you ignore the warning signal or you go too hard for too long, you will lose consciousness for a few seconds.'

Before that, though, there's grey-out, then tunnel vision, and a terrifying six seconds or so of complete blindness where the pilot remains conscious. Then comes A-LOC – 'almost loss of consciousness', which is the point at which g-force starts to affect mental faculties. Symptoms include loss of short-term memory, difficulty in forming words, and trouble with hearing. 'The pilot can generally see and hear, but doesn't care about or adequately attend to what they are seeing and hearing,' according to David Newman in *Flying Fast Jets*. Symptoms can last for up to 20 seconds – more than enough time to get into trouble in a fast-moving aircraft.

Aerobatic pilot Art Scholl once described a case of G-LOC he suffered when completing a vertical figure of eight. He imagined he heard the sound of an alarm clock, and had a vague sense of urgency and that there was something important he had to do. When he regained full consciousness, he was flying upside down, a mile away from the practice area.

Although there have been multiple examples of G-LOC-related deaths in the military context, and the occasional scare around whether rollercoasters could cause brain damage by the same mechanism, in a sporting context things are pretty safe. In the Red Bull Air Race, the g-force is monitored and pilots are disqualified if they exceed 10 g. In fact, in Gdynia, Canadian pilot Pete McLeod is disqualified as he goes over 11 g making the steep banked turn that links the two sections of the lap.

Lamb plays down the risks. 'The moment you lose consciousness you would relax, so the g-force is immediately going to go away because the plane is designed that way. It's not going to stay with the g. The moment you let go of the controls, the g goes away and you come back.'

He's had experience. 'Twice,' he recalls. 'Once, intentionally, as a rather naive student flying jets. I went to 25,000 or 30,000 feet and deliberately did it to see what it was like. It was not great. I didn't enjoy it at all. The second time was again in a jet with an instructor, and he just pulled a whole load of g without me expecting it. It's always much better to be the person applying the g because then you know when it's coming and you adapt.

'It took a little bit of a while to be sharp again,' he says. 'I was kind of OK but I just wasn't reacting. My brain felt OK, but my body took a few seconds to react properly.'

There are ways to mitigate against G-LOC, as Lamb explains. 'You need to restrict the flow of blood down your body. I'm quite lucky in my plane because I'm in a very reclined seating position, which reduces the vertical distance between my heart and my brain, so it makes the job easier for my heart to keep the blood up there. And my legs are quite high – they're elevated so the ease of fluid flowing downwards is already restricted a bit. What we do then is we pressurise the chest cavity.'

He puffs out his chest to show me how. 'Huge breath – big, deep breath. Hold your breath. Then squeeze your abdominal, thigh and calf muscles, and then you breathe with just 10 per cent of your lung capacity.' He exhales in short, sharp bursts. 'You just take these short breaths so you keep breathing while keeping the pressure in your chest cavity. You just keep squeezing and relaxing, squeezing and relaxing. It's quite straightforward.'

To make it even easier, the pilots have to wear a g-suit – a skintight contraption that contains four 'fluid muscles' which help pressurise the lower half of the body. It works a bit like a compression bandage you might put on if you sprain your ankle, but on a much grander scale, and it reacts to the compressing movements the pilots make with their own muscles.

'I absolutely hate it,' says Lamb. 'It's restrictive, it's heavy, it's uncomfortable and it's very hot. If you're in Malaysia and it's 38 degrees with high humidity, it's just desperate. And it weighs 6.5 kilos exactly. I've told them to measure mine and make sure it doesn't weigh a gram more than the book figure.'

Still, whether the pilots like them or not, they're fortunate that the sport takes place in an environment where potentially dangerous G-LOC can almost always be prevented, with the right techniques to keep the brain supplied with the oxygen it needs to function.

Nut Cracking

In other sports, such as Formula 1, dealing with g-force is more about endurance. During a normal race, the forces drivers have to contend with are much lower – around 6 g at most – but they will be sustained for longer and repeated every lap for up to two hours. It's incredibly exhausting, both physically and mentally, and there is even some evidence that g-force can affect the way you perceive the positioning of your limbs, which could make driving a car quite tricky if you allow it to interfere.

That's why F1 drivers have to put such an emphasis on muscle strengthening, particularly their necks. Ferrari driver Fernando Alonso's neck muscles are so developed from training that he can crack a walnut with them. Former Red Bull driver Mark Webber described the sensation of g-force in an F1 car, which is different from a plane as it is at a right angle to the body. 'G-force makes it feel as though your body is being squeezed. In a fast corner, the g-force comes on laterally as we go around, so your ribs, hip and neck get squeezed into the edge of the seat. You've got to get used to that. The force comes on slowly and peaks in the middle of the corner.' There's also g-force at play when decelerating. 'That feeling is completely different,' continued Webber in an interview with the *Telegraph*. 'You hit the brakes very, very hard, so the g-force is extremely high but goes away quickly.'

The sharp, sudden application of high g-forces can be extremely damaging to both body and brain. American drag racer Don Garlits, considered the father of his sport, was forced to retire when he braked so sharply during testing that both his retinas detached, leaving his sight at risk. 'It was a terrible, violent stop,' said Garlits, who was nicknamed 'Big Daddy'. 'I pulled the 'chutes at about 250mph and went 166mph through the traps and turned off at the first turn. That son of a gun stopped on a dime and gave me nine cents change. I saw some stars like you do when you get a jolt, but that evening I began to see these flashes.'

In 2003, Swedish driver Kenny Brack was competing in an IndyCar race at the Texas Motor Speedway. With 12 laps to go, his car locked wheels with Tomas Scheckter's, and was flung into the catch fencing that protects spectators from debris. The g-force recorded by the in-car system peaked at 214 g, the highest ever recorded in the sport. Brack fractured his sternum and femur, shattered a vertebra and crushed his ankles. It took him 18 months to recover.

With those kinds of forces at play, it's no wonder that the brain is at risk too. A study looking at the Indy Racing League found that drivers involved in an impact of 50 g or higher had a 16 per cent chance of a head injury. Athletes in other sports routinely subject their heads to even higher g-forces, and without the crumple zones and roll bars that protect racing drivers. Hard hits in sports like American football can exert forces that exceed 100 g, and as we'll see in the next chapter, the effects on the brain can be devastating.

CHAPTER ELEVEN

DEATH BY INDUSTRIAL DISEASE

Chris Nowinski was the first ever Harvard graduate to wrestle in the WWE. The 37-year-old from Illinois majored in sociology, and played as a defensive tackle in the esteemed university's American football team. He didn't make it into the NFL, but after a spell of working as a researcher in the healthcare industry, the six-foot-five tall Nowinski decided to put his athletic abilities to good use and try out for the larger-than-life world of professional wrestling.

'I thought I would hate it, but I fell in love with it,' he said, recalling how he first got into the sport when he was forced to watch it with his college roommates in the small apartment they shared. 'You had to create a character and then tell a story in each match. There were good guys and bad guys, and the arc of a story with a beginning, middle and end.'

Nowinski's character was a bad guy. His persona was 'Chris Harvard', an arrogant, privileged snob whose outfit consisted of spandex briefs with the Harvard 'H' emblazoned on the back. He would routinely play up to his character by taunting and belittling the intelligence of his opponents, and the audience. 'Sometimes I would recite poetry from the ring,' he recalled in his book, *Head Games*. There are other examples, highlighting the absurdity of the WWE in its glory years. 'In a Hardcore match in Bridgeport, Connecticut, I assaulted Al Snow with a human skeleton, ripped off the skull, got down on bended knee, and began reciting Hamlet: "Alas, poor Yorick!"'

In 2003, an incident in the ring sparked a dramatic career change, as Nowinski explains when I speak to him on the phone from his office in Boston. 'I received a concussion wrestling in a non-televised match, in front of about 5,000 people,' he recalls. 'I was supposed to get kicked in the head and I was just too close to the kick, and it caught me under the chin. I immediately forgot where I was, what we were doing.

'My head was throbbing. But I didn't know enough to stop, so we ended up finishing the match, and making up a new ending. Then I went backstage and kind of downplayed my symptoms to the athletic trainer, and even though I had headaches and nausea for weeks I kept on telling the medical team I was fine. I thought I was supposed to tough my way through those sorts of symptoms.' Nowinski continued to perform for over a month afterwards. 'After five weeks I was honest after a night where I was sleepwalking, and injured myself jumping off the bed into the nightstand,' he tells me.

The incident changed his life. 'The headaches were pretty consistent for five years. The sleep disorder lasted for three and a half years – I would act out my dreams, I would have dreams that I was choking to death, other weird things. I had memory problems that lasted for about a year and a half that were pretty tough to deal with, and the depression that you can imagine would come with all those symptoms. I had trouble remembering certain people's names, appointments. I had trouble laying down new memories.'

His epiphany came when, with his symptoms refusing to budge, he visited Dr Robert Cantu, a world-leading concussion expert who happened to be based nearby. Nowinski, who had considered the kick to the head his first ever concussion, was shocked to learn that 'headaches, confusion, dizziness, double vision, or ringing in your ears' were all symptoms too. 'He was the first person to really explain that the "dings" and "bell ringers" were concussions as well,' he says. He was diagnosed with 'post-concussive syndrome' and, to his alarm, he discovered that he was far from alone.

Since then, Nowinski has become an activist in the fight for greater awareness and education about concussion, as well as preventative measures, particularly in youth sports. He set up the Concussion Legacy Foundation (formerly Sports Legacy Institute), a not-for-profit organisation that helps research the dangers of sporting concussion, and lobbies for rule changes.

So far in the book, we've looked at how neuroscience is helping athletes improve. But as well as training the brain to make it better, our increasing knowledge of the brain is also revealing how sport can have a detrimental effect on mental function. Repeated head impacts are affecting athletic performance, and, more importantly, are causing critical long-term problems later in life. Concussions could be the biggest storm to hit contact sport, well, ever – it could change the way you play your favourite sports, or put their very future in jeopardy. If you play American football, rugby or even football, it's important to know the facts so you can make an informed decision about how much risk you're willing to accept.

In 2006, Nowinski published *Head Games: Football's Concussion Crisis,* which has since been made into a documentary of the same name. Now, part of his job is persuading the families of former athletes to donate their loved one's brain tissue to the 'brain bank' – a research lab at Boston University – so that it can be studied.

Breaking Point

In a head impact, the brain gets momentarily squashed out of shape by the extreme g-forces. It twists. This stretches the axons, the long trunks and branches of nerve cells that carry the information that makes the whole thing work. They can handle a slow stretch, but like a piece of Blu-Tack, if you stretch them quickly, they'll snap. It's the speed of the stretch that matters, as Dr Doug Smith, director of the Center for Brain Injury and Repair at the University of Pennsylvania, explained: 'The rapid stretch doesn't break the nerve fibres, but it can damage parts of those nerve fibres. They're like a garden hose, and inside are railroad tracks called micro-tubules that transport material back and forth throughout the axon. And if you break the railroad tracks, all transport stops. It's like the train car just fell off the tracks and everything can pile up.'

Concussion is not just a problem in elite sport. There are between 4 and 5 million sporting concussions a year, according to some estimates. Symptoms range from light-headedness, loss of balance and fatigue, through to memory loss or seizure. A concussion doesn't necessarily involve losing consciousness. Nowinski argues that as many as 80 per cent of concussions in contact sports such as American football or rugby are going undiagnosed, either because players are unaware of the symptoms, or because they're reluctant to show weakness.

A survey of players in the Canadian Football League found between 10 and 40 times more concussions in an anonymous survey than were found when the players had to fill in their names. Two studies into high schoolers found that the reported incidence of concussions varied from 15 per cent to 47 per cent when the better understood term 'head injuries' was used in the question instead of 'concussion', which many people think requires you to be knocked out. The NFL's definition of a concussion is in fact much broader: 'A traumatically induced alteration in brain function manifested by an alteration of awareness or consciousness.'

The day after my media flight in Poland, I pay a visit to the ramshackle home of the Gdynia Seahawks, the town's American football team. In a few weeks, they'll be competing in the Polish American Football League's equivalent of the Super Bowl, so they've gathered the media already in town for the Air Race to try to drum up some interest. There's a distinctly amateurish air to proceedings. The hybrid pitch is in good condition, but there are fewer than a dozen people assembled in the first few rows of the single stand that lines one side of the ground. To the right, a cleaner scrapes bird mess off the concrete steps of the stand with a mop, while below, the commissioner of the league gives a short, poorly prepared presentation. Halfway through, the backboard featuring the logos of the league's various sponsors falls down.

The Seahawks squad is comprised of local players, with a sprinkling of American imports. It's easy to see who is who. The Polish players don't look like athletes at all, while the four Americans are all black, young and bulging with muscle. They're journeymen. Cast adrift by the NFL because of injury or lack of ability, they spend six months at a time in Europe as mercenaries, in places like Finland, Poland, the Czech Republic, before returning home in the close season. It's not glamorous, but they get to do what they love.

As the team practise booting the ball between the posts and throwing it half the length of the field, I spot an opportunity to see whether Nowinski's assertions that athletes don't really know when they've been concussed holds true at this level.

'I've never had a concussion in my life,' insists Lance Kriesien, the team's imposing quarterback, which seems hard to believe. He points me and my dictaphone towards Tunde Ogun, a charismatic running back from Virginia with shoulder-length dreadlocks who is nicknamed 'Nightmare'. He tells me to look up why on YouTube.

When he's back in the States with his young family, Ogun manages a gym and has the biceps to show it. 'I've had three concussions in football games that I was aware of,' he tells me. 'There's no telling the ones you're not aware of.' His experience of the immediate effects is fairly typical. 'The first time I knew I had a concussion, I had temporary hearing loss for a second. I got up, and I couldn't hear anything. I was just watching lips move, so I knew something was wrong. I heard the high-pitched buzzing, my face began to get warm, all those kinds of things.'

In his brain, nerve cells were twisted, and axons had been bent and broken.

Deflector Shields Down

'If you disconnect these axons they're gone forever,' says Smith in *Head Games*. 'You can function without quite a few axons, but at a certain point you're at a disadvantage.' We're born with billions of neurons, many more than we need, and as we develop, the number of connections in the brain actually reduces sharply through a process called 'pruning'.

This is part of the reason why it's harder to learn a new language when you get older, but it also means that the skills we do develop are more streamlined within the brain as we learn. Still, there's always a degree of neural plasticity. If one area of the brain gets damaged, other parts can change and adapt to take over those functions. However, concussions can take out thousands or hundreds of thousands of connections at once, and it's thought that the post-concussive syndrome that Nowinski was diagnosed with could be down to a loss of neural plasticity. After a certain amount of damage, the brain simply runs out of spare capacity and can't cope. A motorway can only cope with so many lanes being closed before things grind to a halt.

This loss of spare brain capacity could also explain why athletes who have suffered a concussion are more likely to have a second one, and why they are between four and seven times more likely to be knocked unconscious. As far as the brain goes, what doesn't kill you definitely doesn't make you stronger.

Welsh rugby player George North received four blows to the head in the space of five months in 2015, and was out of match action for a total of five months, so he has first-hand experience of some of the more lasting symptoms of concussion. 'Something wasn't right,' he says. 'Rugby players are creatures of habit. I'm used to doing four sessions a day, flat out, as hard as I can go, go home, feel tired, and do the same the next day. When I first did it, I would not even do a full session – even just a light session on a bike or something – and I'd go home, sleep all afternoon and be tired. Then I'd make some food and wash the dishes and I'd have a headache from washing the dishes. Little things like that tell you that you're not quite right.'

Symptoms such as memory loss are caused by a change in the chemical balance of the brain after a concussion. As we've seen, neurons communicate with each other by releasing chemicals called neurotransmitters, which are released by one neuron and bind to receptors on the next. These receptors work like canal locks; they open channels or activate pumps in the walls of neurons, changing their chemical balance and triggering them to 'fire'.

This firing releases more neurotransmitters at the other end of the neuron, which then trigger more neurons. Think of a line of beacon towers, like the ones that were used to warn of an invading army: when one tower lights up, the next one along follows, passing the message along quickly over great distances.

In a concussion, too much of a neurotransmitter called glutamate binds to receptors, letting in too much calcium and letting out too much potassium. This chemical imbalance affects the neuron's ability to turn glucose into energy, and the supply of glucose is also interrupted because of decreased blood flow to the brain after a concussion, so the overall effect is a sharp drop in neural connectivity.

The overall effect within the brain is a bit like trying to text your friends on New Year's Eve – the messages aren't going through because there isn't enough bandwidth to go around, and even if you do get through, your friends are in no fit state to react to the information anyway.

Even after the initial symptoms have faded, the damaged cells teeter on the brink, like buildings damaged in an earthquake and vulnerable to aftershocks. If there's another concussion during a window afterwards, there's a real risk of severe permanent damage or death. This is called 'second impact syndrome' and Nowinski likens it to 'the Death Star in the movie *Star Wars* when the deflector shield is down'.

Second impact syndrome is rare but devastating; it mainly affects teenagers. Another hit in the next days, weeks or months can cause death or permanent brain damage in minutes, even if it's just a hit to the chest that jerks the head slightly. There have been cases of young athletes taking a blow to the head, returning days or weeks later, and then collapsing on the field after a minor incident. There's also evidence of even longer-lasting effects from just one concussion – evidence suggests that the risk of suicide can be elevated for up to a year.

Multiple concussions over the course of a career can be equally devastating.

Brains in Boxes

Dave Duerson was desperate to get a message across. He had played defensive back in the NFL for the Chicago Bears, the New York Giants and the Phoenix Cardinals in the late 1980s and early 1990s, winning two Super Bowl titles. On 17 February 2011, though, all his energies were focused on his final communications. He sent a text message to his ex-wife, and hastily scrawled a note which was found later in his Florida apartment. Both carried the same message: 'Please see that my brain is given to the NFL's brain bank.'

Then he shot himself in the chest.

His brain ended up on the autopsy table of Dr Bennet Omalu, the Nigerian physician who first discovered a link between multiple concussions and brain injury. It all started with Pittsburgh Steelers center Mike Webster, whose brain endured the hard hits and tough tackles of a 15-year NFL career, and ended up, without pomp or ceremony, in a plastic tub in Omalu's living room.

Webster was a Pittsburgh hero, although for Omalu, who had little interest in American football, he was merely a local character – he'd heard about his increasingly bizarre behaviour on local news reports.

When he died of a heart attack at the age of 50, the once-revered Webster was homeless, living in a truck with bin bags taped over the windows. Omalu was tasked with performing the autopsy, and he went into it determined to find out what had caused the player's mental deterioration. There was nothing outwardly wrong with Webster's brain, even after Omalu deftly removed it from his skull; but he wanted to take a closer look, and so broke with protocol and the wishes of his colleagues by requesting a microanalysis of slices of the brain. He funded this analysis with his own money, which is why Webster's brain ended up in his living room and not at the morgue.

When the stained slides came back, Omalu was stunned by what he saw: dark brown and red splotches all over Webster's brain tissue. For the first time, he had concrete evidence – from inside a player's brain – that the hard hits endured by NFL players could be the cause of their mental health problems. The disease he had discovered is called 'chronic traumatic encephalopathy', or 'CTE'.

Duerson's brain also tested positive for CTE, which has been implicated in the mental decline and suicide of several other athletes. There's Andre Waters, who played safety for the Philadelphia Eagles. His policy on concussions was to just keep playing. 'I think I lost count at 15,' he said. 'In most cases, nobody knew it but me. I just wouldn't say anything.'

After retirement he began to change, and showed signs of depression, fairly common in retired athletes who miss the glitz and the glamour of professional sport. But he also displayed short-term memory problems and bizarre and worrying behaviour. A friend visited his house and found Waters crying and pleading: 'I need help, somebody help me.'

At the age of 44, Waters shot himself in the head.

The brain lab also found CTE in the brain of Justin Strzelczyk, a former offensive lineman for the Pittsburgh Steelers. He too exhibited strange behaviour shortly after retirement. On the morning of 30 September 2004 he caused a minor traffic accident but fled the scene.

When the police found him, he refused to pull over, throwing bottles at them and leading them on a high-speed chase for 40 miles. For the last three miles he crossed on to the wrong side of the highway, and died when he drove into a tractor trailer at nearly 90 miles an hour.

Chris Benoit was a professional wrestler who, over the course of three days in June 2007, murdered his wife and young son, before hanging himself from a weights machine. According to Nowinski, who was his friend and colleague at the WWE, Benoit was known for his toughness, and had once told him that he had suffered more concussions than he could count. 'He had advanced CTE,' writes Nowinski in an updated version of *Head Games*. 'Whatever role steroids may have played in the situation, I believe he would never have become a murderer without the brain disease.'

When Omalu first published his results in 2005, the NFL tried its hardest to discredit him. The scandal and scale of their attempted cover-up are enough to fill another book, and are the focus of the recent movie *Concussion*, in which Omalu is played by Will Smith.

The league convened its own medical panel, declared Omalu's work flawed, and churned out sponsored research casting doubt on the claims of Omalu and others like him. But the evidence continued to pile up. The Boston brain lab looked at 34 brains of deceased players and found evidence of CTE in 33 of them. Another study, commissioned by the NFL itself and leaked to the press, surveyed over a thousand players and found that those aged 50 and over were five times more likely than the rest of the US population to be diagnosed with 'dementia, Alzheimer's disease, or other memory-related disease', and that those between the ages of 30 and 49 were 19 times more likely.

The NFL has been slowly waking up to the longer-term dangers of repeated concussions over the course of a career, as tests on the brains of more and more players come back positive for CTE. In April 2015, a US judge awarded $900m in damages to more than 5,000 retired NFL players who accused the league of wilfully hiding the dangers of concussion.

Punch-Drunk

In a small room at Glasgow's Southern General hospital, Dr Willie Stewart extracts a long cardboard box from a shelf stacked with them. I'm expecting it to contain index cards or other documents, something to match the thick volumes of journals and other papers that fill the room.

Stewart is one of the world's leading experts on traumatic brain injury, and as a rugby fan he's been particularly vocal about the need for sport to change. The box he pulls out isn't filled with yellowing cards or files – it contains slices of brain, encased in paraffin wax. There are thousands of samples, from over 40 years of research into traumatic brain injury and its effects. 'Nowhere else in the world can access material like this,' says Stewart, a Glasgow native.

There are other rooms, along a pristine corridor in this new multimillion-pound hospital. One hums with the noise of chest freezers, some of which contain blood and DNA samples for other departments; four of them are full of brain samples waiting to be analysed. In another room, which smells strongly of formaldehyde, a couple of anatomy students watch one of Stewart's colleagues preparing slices of brain for examination under a microscope.

'To me, it looks like the brain essentially starts to rot once you get too many hits, and it just keeps on going,' says Nowinski when I ask him to describe what CTE looks like in the brain. 'The most advanced case of CTE was a former NFL running back whose brain had shrunk to half its original size when he died.'

All cells, neurons included, are made up of complex arrangements of proteins. CTE is triggered when concussive forces disrupt the protein skeleton of nerve fibres. The nerve cells try to rebuild but, after multiple hits, they slowly lose the ability to hold their proteins together. These 'tau proteins' are meant to stabilise the microtubules (the railroad tracks of the neuron mentioned earlier) and, when they malfunction, the tubes collapse, impairing brain function.

Then, the clumps of anomalous tau protein from these collapsed tubes start getting redistributed abnormally in the brain, taking on different shapes and forms called neurofibrillary tangles within brain cells.

There's also another protein called amyloid, which has been found in former athletes with impaired mental function. No one is quite sure what amyloid does, but it is transported down the rail tracks of the microtubules and, when they break in a concussion, amyloid comes crashing off them. 'It's a bit like derailing a cargo train – you get tons of the stuff building up,' says Stewart.

In his office, Stewart takes out some sample slides of confirmed cases of CTE to show me under the microscope. The first one is a footballer. We're looking at a small vertical slice through the brain – through the hippocampus, which is involved in the encoding of long-term memories, among other things. The slides have been treated with a dye that sticks to the abnormal tau protein, so it shows up red against the white and grey matter of the brain.

Healthy areas of the brain treated in this way are a kind of translucent white; they have a marbled look, like an expensive floor. This footballer's brain is stained red. Abnormal tau looks like bloodstains on the marble, and there are smaller dark flecks of brown in certain areas. 'That cluster of brown stains is all that is left of the hippocampus,' says Stewart. 'Extensive abnormal tau.'

The second brain he shows me belonged to a rugby player. The staining comes in bands – at the heart of the brain it's less damaged, but as you go nearer the surface there's a layer of abnormal staining. It's the opposite pattern to that seen in Alzheimer's disease. Abnormal tau and amyloid proteins are also a feature of that degenerative brain disease, but in Alzheimer's the tangles appear in the deeper layers of the brain, while in CTE they're closer to the surface.

Some of the symptoms are the same: CTE can cause cognitive impairment, Parkinsonism, a loss of co-ordination and balance, and behavioural change, as well as emotional control and memory problems. There's a harrowing example of the latter in a clip from the *Head Games* documentary, in which Dr Cantu tests Gene Atkins, a former safety for the New Orleans Saints and Miami Dolphins. First he asks him to repeat the digits '9-7-8-4-3-2', but Atkins can only remember the first three. Then, he asks him to say the months of the year in order.

ATKINS: 'January, February . . . April.'
CANTU: 'Say them in order, like: January, February, March, April . . .'
ATKINS: 'January, February, March, April . . . June.'
CANTU: 'What comes before June?'
ATKINS: '. . . July?'

It's thought that, like in Alzheimer's, abnormal tau can spread through the brain in CTE. In American football players, it tends to move from the prefrontal cortex (involved in decision-making) to the temporal lobes and the hippocampus, which is involved in memory and learning, and then the amygdala, which controls emotion and the flight, fight or freeze response.

Stewart is keen to stress that the relationship between tau and amyloid protein build-up and the symptoms of CTE is as yet unclear; he's not sure whether they cause the problems, or are simply a symptom of them. There have been attempted treatments for Alzheimer's which have successfully tried to clear amyloid proteins from the brain, but haven't actually had any effect on brain function. 'It may be because of other stuff happening in the brain causing the problem,' says Stewart. 'Damage to the axons, the blood-brain barrier breaking down, inflammation.'

CTE is, of course, not just a problem for American football. Other sports have suspected a link between head impacts and mental issues for decades. A paper from 1928 looked into 'punch-drunk' boxers, calling the disease 'dementia pugilistica' and noting symptoms such as slow movement, tremors, confusion and speech problems. They will all be familiar to anyone who has seen Muhammad Ali struggle with Parkinson's disease in the last few decades. Like CTE, it's an affliction common in boxers.

A study of UK boxers found a link between symptoms of CTE and career length. A quarter of those with a career that lasted longer than a decade showed symptoms, while other research has found that increasing the number of matches, knockouts and punches taken also increases the risk.

It's not just CTE either. Concussions have been linked to other brain diseases that can strike in a matter of years rather than decades. Motor neurone disease is a devastating neurodegenerative ailment that kills most sufferers within five years because they lose the ability to control their breathing. Symptoms include muscle spasticity, and difficulty speaking and swallowing. It's also known as amyotrophic lateral sclerosis (ALS), but in the United States it's most commonly referred to as Lou Gehrig's disease, after the celebrated baseball player who died from it at the age of 37. The incidence of ALS is higher in athletes than the general population, and there's growing evidence that it can be triggered or worsened by concussions.

In 1939, after he was diagnosed, Lou Gehrig made an impassioned speech to a sold-out crowd at the Yankee Stadium, in which he called himself 'the luckiest man on the face of the earth' for the career he had enjoyed.

However, he was desperately unlucky. Although he played a non-contact sport, Gehrig was knocked out several times during his career – by pitches, opponents, and once when he threw a punch and missed during a post-game brawl, hitting his head on concrete. 'Although he had a headache, and his head was so swollen he had to borrow one of Babe Ruth's larger baseball caps, against a doctor's orders he played the next day,' writes Nowinski. Gehrig played 2,130 consecutive games, and the disease that bears his name could have been triggered or accelerated by playing through concussion.

Changing Cultures

Perhaps if Jamie Roberts had been a few more years into his medical degree back in 2008, he wouldn't have played on. There were less than two minutes on the clock at the Millennium Stadium when the Wales centre collided with Australia captain Stirling Mortlock in a sickening clash of heads.

'I actually suffered a fractured skull, but the doctor came on the pitch, assessed me, I felt OK to carry on, he was happy for me to play on and you always trust your doctors,' he says. 'He was happy for me to carry on playing, but it was only 10 or 15 minutes later, I felt my symptoms getting worse and signalled to the doctor that I had to go off.'

That's a common theme in some of the athletes worst affected by CTE – they would play on through their concussions. Along with the threat of second impact syndrome, this is why it's so dangerous when athletes return to the field of play too soon after a concussion.

It's in the culture of certain sports to try to play down injuries, to brush them off and carry on, and concussions are no exception to that. 'You can't play the game worried about a concussion because then you're not playing the game at the speed or the level that it's supposed to be played,' says Ogun. 'It's just one of the things I think comes with the territory. I mean, you don't join the military thinking about "am I gonna get shot?" – it's part of the job. If it happens, it happens. It's the same thing with football, you know, it's a high-intensity game, high level. Guys are gonna come at you.'

Nowinski is keen to educate athletes on the dangers. 'Concussions regularly cause problems with balance, reaction time and cognition,' he says. 'So what I tell athletes is that they're usually dumber and slower when they're on the field, and they become a liability for the team. And I think the World Cup in Brazil showed that – a couple of players who played through concussion were only pulled when they made a mistake that exposed the team to a near goal, so that's what the athletes should also be told. They should come off not only because it's the right thing for their health, but also because it's the right thing for their team.'

Attitudes are changing, according to Roberts, who is now a fully trained doctor after completing his medical degree in 2013. 'Go back six or seven years, and there were players – not just in the professional game but down to the amateur game – who would get knocked out, go to the side of the pitch, have a splash of cold water on their face and go back on. It's that macho, bravado side of, "Yeah, I got knocked out but I'll carry on playing."

'People are slowly getting there,' he continues. 'But it's not just the players who need to be educated – it's coaches, parents and referees. It's everyone outside the game who can take decisions away from players. If I was a player playing for a team on a Saturday and I got knocked out for my local club ... You want to carry on playing and go back to training Tuesday ready for next Saturday. It's important for that decision to be taken out of players' hands, and that's where coaches and coach education is paramount in making sure players are safe before they return to play.'

On that front, things are moving in the right direction. The Premier League implemented new rules on concussions at the start of the 2014/15 season after a few high-profile incidents in which players who had been knocked unconscious returned to the field of play. The changes include a neutral concussion doctor in the tunnel to determine whether a player should return. They've also introduced baseline testing, a system already in use in the NFL and in rugby. Players receive a series of tests at the start of the season designed to assess their mental sharpness, and then after a suspected concussion they'll be tested again to see if there's been any change before being allowed back. There are a number of companies offering computerised baseline testing for concussion assessment – programmes include imPACT and CogSport (COG for short).

Technology is also helping the testing, and head injury assessment as a whole, become more efficient and effective. CSx, a New

Zealand-based company, has created an app called Head Guard, which brings together the various assessments and cognitive tests into one interface. 'It's a tool to help doctors make an informed decision,' CEO Ed Lodge tells me on a trip to England during the 2015 Rugby World Cup. 'With the World Cup, you've got independent doctors conducting these tests and they don't necessarily know the players – they shouldn't know them at all – so having the baseline on hand gives the match-day doctors real-time data to enable them to make an informed decision on whether the person has a discrepancy to their normal.' This is particularly useful for pitch-side assessments which are used when the medical staff aren't sure whether a player is concussed or not. In the heat of the match, instead of flicking through printed sheets of questions and forms, they can simply press some buttons on a tablet computer.

The app also brings together all the players' previous tests and assessments for both club and country, and syncs with online storage so it's accessible from anywhere. Plus it can be used for tracking symptoms as players recover and await a return to play. CSx want their technology to be rolled out to the whole professional game, and are also creating a lightweight version that can be used by amateur players. With the Head Guard software able to track players' previous scores and which questions they've been asked in the past on baseline tests, it can help mitigate one of the biggest problems with baseline testing. Players can, and do, game the system.

Former Scotland international Rory Lamont suffered dozens of concussions during his rugby career, and insists players know how to cheat the baseline testing system and return to play when they shouldn't. 'Players can view the baseline test as an obstacle in their way for getting back playing,' he wrote in an article for ESPN.co.uk. 'To achieve an accurate score, you must pay full attention. The conflict of interest is this: the better score you set in the baseline test, the more difficult it will be to pass the test after concussion. Set a high score and you might end up missing more games than you would like; put in 80 per cent effort and it will be easier to pass the COG test after concussion. Players will deliberately cheat the protocol by putting in a sub-maximal effort when setting their baseline. Without maximum concentration and effort, the COG test will be unreliable for identifying if a player is suffering concussive symptoms.'

Stewart agrees that current baseline tests are flawed. 'None of that stuff is reliable enough,' he tells me. 'The current testing that's available across sports has a reliability, in good hands, of 70-85 per cent, maximum. Which means you're talking about anywhere between 15 to 30 per cent of concussions being missed. That's not a good enough value. Players who have been unconscious have managed to pass the available test.'

He shows me what he thinks is a better baseline test, one that can't really be cheated. The King-Devick test is very simple: it's a series of flashcards, each of which contains rows of numbers. The player has to read out the numbers from top to bottom and left to right as quickly as possible. The cards get progressively harder. In the first one, there are lines to guide the eye, but later on the numbers get squashed together or placed in positions where it's hard to see what row they're in. Doing the test multiple times in quick succession makes it harder to cheat, because if a player tries to go deliberately slowly they won't be able to match that time the second or third time they do it, whereas if they go as fast as they can, like they're supposed to, their times will remain very similar.

It also works a variety of different areas of the brain. 'Seeing the number – visual cortex, saying the number out loud – speech cortex, and at the same time you're trying to move on to the next number,' says Stewart. 'All of that is the longest pathways inside your brain you could possibly come up with. Back to front, front to back, side to side – a whole bunch of very long pathways and they're all in the right place for rotational injury. Somebody being tested with a brain injury on this ends up three, four, five, six, 10 seconds slower than he was.'

Other ways of detecting head injuries in sport have also been explored. After George North's double concussion against England, rugby's governing body suggested the use of video – monitoring play for incidents and impacts the touchline doctors may have missed.

Another way of spotting and understanding concussions could be through the use of sensors – measuring and tracking the g-forces that players' heads are subjected to during play. There are a number of helmet-bound sensors that can be used for American football, although the NFL are yet to adopt any. 'There are a lot of variables we don't understand about why one hard hit will cause concussion and one hard hit won't,' Nowinski tells me. 'There's a lot of suspicion that it's rotational acceleration – the twisting.'

CSx have developed a sensor for rugby which can be worn behind the ear, applied with skin-safe adhesive or tucked under a scrum cap, to measure head movement in real time. It's early days, but Lodge and colleagues plan to examine head movement, video evidence and subsequent symptoms to determine what kind of movements trigger concussion. Their system records data over 3,000 times a second. 'We get a high-definition picture of the impact,' says Lodge. 'We're looking to build a risk index. There isn't going to be a number that can diagnose concussion, and a sensor should never diagnose concussion. What it is really about is giving information to the medics or people on the sidelines. We're developing an algorithm based on the linear movement and rotation.'

Another sensor, which is currently being trialled across the US, is the Linx IAS headband, which has its origins in the military where it was tested as a way of measuring shockwaves from explosive blasts – giving medics an assessment of the potential severity of damage to a soldier's brain. The sensor is a fabric headband, rather than being fitted to a helmet, and reports blows wirelessly on a scale from one to 99. Another technology, called FITGuard, builds the sensor into a mouthguard which players wear.

The idea is that this technology could be used as an early warning system for head injuries – not to diagnose whether or not a player needs to come off, but just to flag whether they should be looked at.

There's an argument that this data, and the use of head-injury tracking software, should become mandatory, and should be in the hands of the authorities rather than individual teams. If an independent doctor in the NFL or rugby had access to video footage, head movement data and a player's baseline test scores, they would be better placed to make an impartial call in that player's best interests. Until then, though, while players are more educated now than ever, some will still put their brains on the line to stay on the pitch.

Death by Industrial Disease

The dry language of the coroner's report boiled down Jeff Astle's career of crashing headers into four words: death by industrial disease. There is compelling evidence that even less powerful 'sub-concussive' impacts could lead to CTE and other brain damage. Astle, who played as a striker for West Brom and England in the 1960s and 1970s, passed away in 2002, originally diagnosed with Alzheimer's disease. But a re-examination of his brain by Dr Stewart found signs of CTE – and his family's Justice for Jeff campaign has fought a battle for recognition from the football authorities in England that heading a heavy leather football contributed to Astle's demise and mental decline.

After his brain came back positive for CTE, Astle's widow Laraine told Sky Sports News: 'We've always known what killed Jeff but now we know 200 per cent. There's no ifs or buts. You find it so hard to believe that football can do that. It's terrible to think what he went through. The job he loved in the end killed him. Everything he won, he remembered none of it.'

Other cases of CTE in former footballers have been identified: Brazil's 1958 World Cup-winning captain Bellini reportedly had grade four CTE (the highest level) when he died, after suffering from symptoms including memory loss in the last years of his life. Once, years after he retired, he hired a taxi to drive him to Sao Paulo FC's base because he thought he had to go to training.

It is not, as some have argued, a problem confined to the old days of heavy leather footballs made weightier still when soaked with rain or caked in mud. American semi-pro Patrick Grange died in 2012 at the age of just 29. He had ALS and grade two CTE. The game has got faster and more powerful since Astle's time, and, even at amateur level, players connect their foreheads to balls travelling in excess of 50 miles an hour, which can weigh half a kilo.

In New York, Michael Lipton and colleagues at the Albert Einstein College of Medicine wanted to see if there was a direct link between heading the ball and damage to the brain in living players. They asked 37 amateur players about how many times they had headed the ball in the previous year, and then put them through a standard cognitive test and scanned their brains with MRI.

There's a (possibly apocryphal) story about former England striker Gary Lineker which suggests that he would refuse to head the ball in training – and some of the participants in this study may have been doing the same thing, because there was a vast range of heading experience. The fewest number of headers completed in the year leading up to the tests was 32, while the highest was 5,400.

There was a link between number of headers and cognitive test scores. Those who had completed more headers did worse, and the white matter of their brains (which coats neurons to speed up signals) had less structural coherence. 'Everything really converged to say that the more heading you did, the worse your brain looked,' said Lipton in an interview with the *New Yorker.* He continued: 'The question is: How different are you than you would be if that had not happened? Or, to make it sound really horrible, let's say you have a twelve-year-old child playing competitive soccer and heading. What is the expected cognitive or behavioural trajectory of that kid? And how is that altered or impeded by this exposure?'

Recent research by Eric Nauman and colleagues at Purdue University, Indiana, followed two high school women's football teams and one college-level team over the course of a season. The players wore a sensor called the xPatch, which tracked the g-force and rotation of impacts to the head, and the researchers also tracked their training sessions, monitoring what kind of impacts caused what kind of forces in a similar way to the work being done in the NFL and rugby. In addition, they took MRI scans of the players' brains before, during and after the season to track how they changed – the first study of its kind looking at the direct impact of sub-concussive impacts on the brain.

They found much higher g-forces than they expected, particularly in players heading the ball back from goal kicks – the high-looping deliveries that drop from the sky created g-force levels similar to a boxer's punch. 'The percentage of 100 g hits was effectively the same between women's college soccer and American football, which really surprised us,' Nauman told the *Guardian*. 'And while American football players tend to take more hits overall in a given practice session and game, the college soccer players were getting hit every day and so it evened out.'

Early analysis of the MRI scans has revealed damage to blood vessels supporting the brain. 'If you actually compare the brains of people who have taken a lot of sub-concussive hits to ones that have taken a single big hit, the sub-concussive brains often look worse,' continued Nauman. 'I don't think people appreciate that yet.'

Other tests have found memory impairments and abnormal brain activity in high school football players who took hard hits during the previous week, but without suffering a concussion. MRI scans of adult football players who had been playing since they were children found loss of white matter in areas of the brain critical to memory, attention and visual processing. They also performed poorly on cognitive tests. Could footballers have a reputation for a lack of intelligence because the sport is actually damaging their brains?

'You can bruise any other part of your body and it feels sore,' said Nauman. 'But when the same thing happens to your brain, it doesn't have the pain receptors to tell you to ease off for a few days. That is enough to really cause problems.'

'Just because you don't have physical symptoms doesn't mean you haven't damaged your brain,' Stewart tells me. There may soon be a way to detect brain damage without physical symptoms, a better measure than baseline tests or g-force sensors, which can never diagnose a concussion with certainty or tell you anything about the extent of the damage. There is a potential blood test for brain damage.

When neurons in the brain die, they release a protein called SNTF. 'When an axon is damaged with no hope of recovery it switches this on as a sort of suicide response, "Sayonara, we're off,"' says Stewart. His lab has recently finished work proving that this protein does come from injured axons, which paves the way for it to be used as a test for concussion – perhaps not by the side of the pitch, but in the days afterwards. 'Say you and I bang heads and we both feel as dazed and we both go along and get a blood test done that day or the next day, and my SNTF is high and your SNTF hasn't changed, you'll be fit to play again in days, whereas I'll be the one who, some days or weeks later, is still struggling to shake their symptoms,' says Stewart.

It's the degree of injury to the axons that predicts how severe symptoms of a concussion will be, and how long it will take to recover from them, and it's the degree of injury to axons that determines longer-term conditions such as CTE. 'What you could do is to take George North the day after the England match and do a blood test on him,' says Stewart. 'George North passed all his concussion tests, but my feeling is you could probably do a blood sample on him and find that actually he may be passing all his subjective concussion tests but deep down his brain has been damaged, and so it doesn't matter what is said, we'll treat him differently.'

The Great Gazoo

Mark Kelso took a lot of stick when he started wearing the ProCap, a layer of padding that fits over the top of an NFL helmet like a soft thimble over a thumb, but he reckons it increased his playing career by several years. 'I took a lot of kidding,' said the Buffalo Bills safety, 'getting called "Bubblehead" and "Gazoo" because of how it looked, but I stopped getting concussions.'

ProCap was found to reduce the force of head-on collisions in American football by 30 per cent, compared to the standard hard-plastic models, but the technology has not been widely adopted. Things are starting to change, though.

Traditional helmet technology in the NFL is beginning to improve. For years, helmets did a great job of protecting the skull from damage, but almost nothing to stop the brain twisting around inside, which is what causes concussion. One study found that although helmets were excellent at stopping skull fractures and external bruising, they only lessened the risk of concussion by 20 per cent on average, while another found big variations between different brands of helmet. Studies have begun to use sensors to try to improve the design of helmets to minimise the risk of concussion. Newer models have introduced increased protection to the side of the head to mitigate against those blows, which are thought to cause more concussions than head-on blows. Among those new approaches is the VICIS helmet, which deforms on impact like a car bumper to reduce the severity of impacts on the brain.

Another method is inspired by woodpeckers. The birds withstand immense forces while drilling their way into trees, and have evolved a unique strategy for protecting their brains: their tongue curls around the inside of their skull, increasing the blood pressure and preventing the brain from moving around inside. It's hoped that a collar which slightly compresses the jugular vein in the throat could have the same effect in humans. 'It creates an artificial air bag, making the brain more solid to the skull,' said Dr Gregory Myer, who is leading the research effort with ice hockey players.

'I remember when I first started playing football when I was six years old, the helmets were so hard,' says Ogun. 'The padding wasn't the same. Nowadays, you put on a helmet and it's like a couch on your head.' He continues: 'But then again it doesn't suffice for the trauma. You got a guy like Lance – he's 250 pounds. If he hits you I don't care what you have on your head, you're gonna feel it. They're taking all the necessary steps, but I don't think it's anything that's ever gonna be fully eliminated. You've just got to play the game the best you can, protect yourself the best you can, and hope for the best.'

Nowinski and others aren't content with that. They believe that changing the game is the only way to make sport safe from the scourge of CTE. Nowinski's Concussion Legacy Foundation has launched a safer soccer programme, which seeks to eliminate heading the ball before high school level. 'I think football, as seen from the World Cup, is far behind,' says Nowinski. 'It's probably the biggest problem in sport – you have the most important and popular sport in the world doing everything wrong on the international stage. It sort of sets the world back.'

In 2014 – after a World Cup competition in which a couple of players played on through obvious concussions – a group of current and former players and the parents of youth players in America launched a class action lawsuit against FIFA and US Soccer, demanding rule changes around the management and prevention of head trauma and concussion. And, in fact, on the morning I speak to Stewart in November 2015, US Soccer announce a ban on heading the ball for players under the age of 13.

'At least 30 per cent of concussions are caused by attempting to head the ball,' Nowinski says. He also advocates the use of a 'Hit Count' – tracking every head impact of greater than 20 g and limiting the exposure of young athletes to sub-concussive impacts. Nowinski is focusing his efforts on youth because that's where the greatest risk is. 'Although kids don't look like they hit each other hard, the sensors tell us they do because they have bigger heads relative to their body and weak necks, so it doesn't take much to accelerate their brain,' he says. 'And, at the same time, they don't have doctors on the sidelines to help them; they're too young to realise when they're hurt and their coaches may not be as well trained.'

There are other ways of reducing the risk. At the start of the 2011 season, the NFL changed the rules on kick-off returns, moving them back from the 30-yard line to the 35-yard line in an attempt to reduce the number of violent, high-speed collisions as the receiving team and kicking team charge towards each other. It seemed to work: according to the NFL's own data, concussions on kick-offs fell by 40 per cent between 2011 and 2012, part of an overall reduction of 13 per cent. There's even talk of removing kick-offs from the game entirely.

Less drastic tweaks could push that figure down further. Heads Up Football is an education programme for coaches and young American football players that aims to teach them about the dangers of concussion – how to recognise and prevent it. It also features Heads Up Tackling, a new way of taking down your opponent that focuses on hitting them with the shoulder instead of the helmet strike which often causes injury.

Another way of reducing the risk of CTE is to remove those most in danger of it from the game entirely. A gene called ApoE4 which has been linked to Alzheimer's has also been implicated in how well an individual can recover from concussion. It's thought to influence how quickly the brain clears itself of amyloid, a protein that builds up after brain injury. Deposits of this protein have been found in 40 to 45 per cent of individuals with CTE.

Boxers with a copy of the ApoE4 gene scored worse on tests of brain impairment than boxers who had similar-length careers but didn't have the gene. Five of the nine American football players with CTE identified by the Boston brain lab in 2009 had the gene – between double and triple the proportion in the general population. Mandatory testing of boxers for the gene has been considered, as a possible way of preventing CTE, or at least identifying those at most risk of developing it, and Stewart thinks it will become widely adopted in sport.

One of the problems is that there's currently no way of assessing CTE in living people. The abnormal tau protein that signals it can only be detected in slices on microscope slides. However, that could soon change. Researchers have recently developed a compound called FDDNP, which attaches to abnormal tau, allowing it to be picked up on a scanner in living people. 'You inject [it] in a vein,' Julian Bailes, one of the researchers, told *USA Today*. 'It circulates through the body. It binds with any tau in the brain, and then you put them inside the scan and you see the picture of it.' In this small pilot study, they examined five former NFL players and found a build-up of tau protein in exactly the same areas in which it has been seen in the autopsied brains of CTE patients.

The surest sign, though, is in the symptoms; and a number of athletes have chosen to cut their careers short after concussions rather than continue playing and risk negative effects in the long term. England rugby player Shontayne Hape retired at 33 after suffering more than 20 concussions during his career. He called it quits when brain scans revealed the extent of damage to his neural function. 'Things got so bad I couldn't even remember my pin number,' he told the *New Zealand Herald*. 'The specialist explained that my brain was so traumatised, had swollen so big, that even just getting a tap to the body would knock me out. I had to retire immediately.'

San Francisco 49ers linebacker Chris Borland retired at just 24, citing fear of concussions as the cause. 'I just honestly want to do what's best for my health,' he told ESPN. 'From what I've researched and what I've experienced, I don't think it's worth the risk.' Borland, who tore up a $3m contract to quit, continued: 'I've thought about what I could accomplish in football, but for me personally, when you read about Mike Webster and Dave Duerson and Ray Easterling [former Atlanta Falcons safety who committed suicide aged 62], you read all these stories, and to be the type of player I want to be in football, I think I'd have to take on some risks that as a person I don't want to take on.

'I just want to live a long, healthy life, and I don't want to have any neurological diseases or die younger than I would otherwise.'

An Unlikely Cure

A glass of red wine is a powerful thing. According to the *Daily Mail*, the drink can help you lose weight, improve your heart health, cut the risk of bowel cancer, *raise* the risk of breast cancer, and ward off symptoms of dementia such as memory loss. It may even be able to undo some of the damage found in CTE. Resveratrol, a compound found in red wine, and the skin of grapes, blueberries and raspberries, has been shown to slow the development of chronic neurodegenerative diseases in animals.

'We know from animal studies that if we give the drug immediately after or soon after a brain injury, it can dramatically and significantly reduce the damage you see long term,' said Dr Joshua Gatson of the University of Texas when launching a pilot study with boxers in 2011. 'The only treatment available is rest and light exercise, but there is no drug therapy to protect the brain from consecutive concussions, which are actually a lot worse than the initial one,' he continued. 'There's been a lot of work with resveratrol showing that it also protects the brain, so we thought this might be the ideal drug.'

Gatson has also found that estrone, one of the body's three naturally occurring oestrogen hormones, can reduce inflammation and cell death after brain injury in mice, possibly by boosting levels of the brain-growth protein BDNF. A range of other substances have potential: curcumin (a compound found in turmeric), creatine, green tea, fish oil, caffeine and vitamins C, D and E are among them.

Another interesting avenue of research is light therapy, in which a powerful beam is shone through the skull and penetrates about a centimetre (half an inch) into the brain, where it's thought to help restore the chemical balance of brain cells. Concussed mice have shown improved brain function after this treatment, and research is ongoing with children and soldiers showing persistent concussion symptoms.

Some clinics are already using such methods and other proprietary substances to try to treat CTE in former athletes and others, but research is yet to prove the effectiveness of these treatments in humans. For desperate families, though, it's a last resort. A bona fide cure would be a real sporting revolution, because, without one, it is unclear whether certain sports have a future in their current form.

Stewart, a sports fan and a doctor, doesn't think it's quite as drastic as that. 'It's one of those difficult balances that somebody is going to have to make. We may find that actually your risk of dementia doubles by playing football or rugby at a high level. But is that a risk worth taking if the flip side is that your risk of cardiovascular disease and diabetes is halved? My fear is that until we get data that we can reliably work with, people give up the sport and then we end up with a bunch of health problems from that.

'I hope in 10 years' time that we've got to a position where it's just seen as culturally abhorrent for people to even consider playing on with brain injury,' he continues. 'And I hope we've got a better idea of what the significance might be long term, so instead of just saying it's a risk for dementia, we'll know it's a doubling of the risk, for example.'

He wants people to be able to make an informed decision. 'People can actually sit down with that information and say, "Well, I want to play rugby. I'll accept the potential increased risk of dementia but I'll balance that against the wonderful benefits of longer life." If we get to that point I think we'll have done a lot.'

There is the potential for even wider good to come out of concussion research. 'The rest of it then is to sit down over the next decades and figure out what the actual physiology of it is, because it's fascinating,' says Stewart. 'I believe that if we can figure out what happens in trauma with degenerating brains, we'll have figured out what happens with degenerating brains full stop. It's the same stuff – blood-brain barrier, inflammatory reaction, tau, amyloid, axons – all that stuff happens in Alzheimer's.'

Concussion is one of the biggest issues in sport, and, as we've seen in this chapter, it's not a problem with an easy solution. Technology is already helping to make sport safer by reducing the risk of concussion, and improving detection and treatment. But, as Stewart explains, working out what happens in an athlete's brain during and after a blow to the head could have far-reaching implications both in sport and beyond.

CHAPTER TWELVE
DOPAMINE JUNKIES

Trollveggen, the Troll Wall, rises up from the valley below like a collection of twisted skyscrapers. Its gnarled tips have an almost gothic air – Gaudi gone mad – with rocky peaks and outcrops stripped bare and whipped into fantastical shapes by the elements. Legend in this part of Norway has it that a group of trolls were on their way back from a wedding celebration, but dawdled too long, and when the first rays of the sun hit them, they were frozen in place to form Trollveggen's individual peaks. The Troll Wall has its place in extreme sports legend too, although the athletes involved were not that interested in the warped rocks themselves, more the sheer drop of more than a mile below them.

Thin cloud grazes the spires of the Troll Wall as Rudy Cassan, Espen Fadnes and five others look across from Romsdalshorn, a slightly kinder looking mountain on the other side of the valley. One of them makes a phone call, and then a few minutes later, four of the group approach the edge together and throw themselves at the ground. I'm watching with around a dozen others from a rocky outcrop further down – but still a steep drive up the 11 hairpin bends of the Trollstigen road, and then a 40-minute scramble uphill for the best vantage point.

It's hard for my brain to process exactly what's going on when they make their exit. I wrote earlier about how the brain uses shortcuts – schema – to make sense of the world around. I have no schema for this. Our first sight of the jumpers is as small dots, like distant birds or planes. They look like glitches on a computer screen, dead pixels in the Norwegian sky. They are BASE jumpers, falling in formation at about 200kph – but from a distance they look like abandoned balloons, drifting slowly towards the ground.

It's only when they get a bit closer that you start to get a real sense of their shape and speed. They're wearing wingsuits, made of a high-tech material that catches the air like a sail. They give the BASE jumpers the ability to glide through the air – to fly, almost. It changes their glide ratio from 1:1 to 2:1 – for every metre they fall, the wingsuit allows them to travel forward two, thanks to a system of air pockets and locks. The noise is the most striking thing about watching these daredevils in person. It's a tearing, ripping noise. It's only the sound of the air flowing past the edges of their suits, but it seems as loud as a jet engine.

It may as well be the sound of the laws of the universe being torn up. This seems utterly impossible – it's the craziest thing I've ever seen – particularly when two of the four jumpers peel out of their formation and perform a banked turn right in front of us. One of them lets out a yell of triumph and delight, and a split second later they've veered away from our collection of dropped jaws, still falling and getting smaller again as they sink into the valley below us.

There are several agonising seconds while we wait for them to pull their parachutes, and then they pop in quick succession – one, two, three, four. The jumpers have enough skill and modern parachutes are so manoeuvrable that they are able to steer them to a soft landing within metres of where they have parked their cars. It is truly amazing – and this is just a routine jump. Online you can see clips of BASE jumpers and wingsuit pilots weaving between buildings, diving into caves, jumping out of helicopters or skiing off the side of mountains.

BASE stands for building, antenna, span and earth. It was coined in a brainstorming session by a group of skydivers who were the pioneers of the sport in the 1970s. They took the concept of freefalling from planes and applied it to tall buildings (B), antenna towers (A), bridges (S) and cliffs or mountains (E). If you complete a jump from each of those four categories you earn a BASE number – around 2,000 people have claimed theirs.

Carl Boenish was BASE #4, but he is considered the father of the sport because of his relentless drive to share its thrills with a larger audience. He created beautiful movies shot with head- and belly-mounted cameras – much heavier equipment than the light and cheap GoPro cameras favoured today. Like all BASE jumpers, he started out in skydiving, but soon craved more. He jumped off El Capitan in Yosemite National Park numerous times, and would engineer ever more outlandish stunts, including one that involved leaping off a bridge from a moving train.

Risk is inherent in this kind of activity, and, alas, there are only so many times the dice can land in your favour. Boenish is #7 on another list. In 1984, he and his wife Jean came to Norway to tackle the Troll Wall, accompanied by a television crew who wanted to film them setting the record for the highest successful BASE jump – 1,800 metres from the top of the Wall.

They made it safely, but the next morning Carl went back to jump again, alone, from another, more difficult site on the Troll Wall. He may have clipped an outcrop on the way down, or his parachute may have failed to open properly. The father of BASE jumping became the seventh person to die from it. Hundreds more have followed. To this day, his reasons for going back remain a mystery – but the pull of the jump is strong.

'I broke my right talus – the main bone in the ankle. My right femur, high up, near the hip. I broke my right wrist. I broke my radial head and now have a radial head replacement in the elbow. And finally I broke my upper arm and damaged my rotator cuff.' At 16, Jamie Flynn joined the Parachute Regiment and spent eight years serving in Iraq and Afghanistan. The army introduced him to skydiving, and he fell in love with BASE jumping. On 30 June 2014, in Turkey, he jumped from a microlite aircraft in his wingsuit. 'Everything was perfect,' he remembers. 'I opened my parachute and started to fly to my landing area. However, it became quickly apparent I wasn't going to make the landing area so I had to pick an alternative. Now, remember we have split seconds to make decisions in this sport. In that split second, I made a wrong decision that I ended up spending the next year paying for.'

Flynn decided to try to land on what he thought was a patch of grass – only the grass was actually just a thin covering for an area of jagged rocks. His right foot got caught between two rocks as he landed, breaking his ankle, and he sustained the other injuries detailed above as he bounced off the ground before coming to a stop. He lay, screaming in agony, on a remote mountainside for 45 minutes before help reached him.

Still, he was determined to carry on jumping. 'When I got told I wouldn't jump again I laughed and told the doctor, "Let's see about that . . ." Admittedly, I didn't know the severity of the injuries at the time but, like most BASE jumpers I've met, I'm incredibly determined. I set the goal to get back to BASE and that's what I did.' Flynn was one of the lucky ones. More than 200 people have died while BASE jumping – due to bad decisions, malfunctioning equipment or sudden gusts of wind. Why risk it?

Dangerous activities have always attracted a brave few, from big-wave surfers to motorcycle racers in the Isle of Man TT. What drives these people to go against every human instinct for self-preservation? What makes them different from people who would never consider jumping off a building or piloting a bike up narrow lanes at hundreds of miles an hour? And is there something within that extreme group that differentiates the people who push things too far from those who manage to stay just the right side of the narrow line between success and death?

It won't surprise you to learn that the answers are all in their heads.

Totally Addicted to BASE

'The special moment is the one when you just push and exit from the rock, because you change from one world to another world,' says Rudy Cassan, after his jump from Romsdalshorn – he was the jumper who flew past closest to our group. Cassan played the role of Boenish for some BASE-jumping shots in the documentary *Sunshine Superman*, which was released in 2015. After he wolfs down some lunch (apparently, risking your life works up quite the appetite), the Frenchman tells me about what's going through his head when he does a jump like the one I've just witnessed.

'I get stressed before most of my jumps because it's a risk. Every jump is a risk. I have done more than 200 BASE jumps but every jump is a risk, so my heart is starting to pump. Before you're jumping you're at about 160 beats per minute. It's like when you run – your body needs to be focused and concentrated.

'You have the stress, you control the stress, you jump and then after you jump you have all the emotions going through you and the endorphins going through your body. If you jump on your own, relaxed, it might not be that much, but if you are with friends or you fly by people you have more energy coming through. It's like an explosion of endorphins when you land. It's definitely addictive, it's not a question,' he says.

Espen Fadnes, another one of the jumpers that day, agrees. 'I'm addicted to adrenaline,' he tells me. 'And that goes through my whole life. I'm never able to keep a relationship; I'm never able to have a normal job. The only stable thing I have in my life is to jump off a mountain with a wingsuit. The rest is just chaos. When I jump off a mountain and I start flying, I feel at peace with myself. I feel like I belong there – and it's a sensation of control, happiness, mastery, and a weird feeling of actually flying. When I land, the normal thought is always towards the next jump – the next shot of adrenaline.'

The supply of adrenaline is controlled by the adrenal glands, which are located above the kidneys. Adrenaline is a powerful stimulant – it's released in times of fear or arousal and fuels the fight, flight or freeze response. It speeds up breathing and heart rate to get more oxygen to the muscles, with the aim of equipping your brain and body to get out of a dangerous situation as quickly as possible. It can feel exhilarating, creating a natural high that can last several hours as the adrenaline clears your system. This is the buzz that 'adrenaline junkies' seek.

The problem is that you quickly become acclimatised to it. Riding a rollercoaster for the first time is thrilling, but if you were to do it every day, your brain would soon learn that it was not a genuine threat and your body would stop releasing adrenaline. You need a bigger and bigger dose of excitement to keep getting the rush. This pushes people to take greater and greater risks in search of that high. 'You have a lot of them,' says Fadnes. 'They start BASE jumping and they take extreme risks. That kind of personality normally quits BASE jumping after a few years because, after a short time, they stop feeling afraid. They stop getting that kick of adrenaline and it becomes boring. Or they die because they are too risk-willing.'

Those who stay alive learn to control their dosage. 'We're willing to step off a mountain,' says Fadnes, 'but we do everything we can to make it as safe as possible. We take small steps forward so that we never lose that feeling of fear and that feeling of adrenaline.'

Most of the people I speak to claim they don't do it for the adrenaline; although their sports are dangerous, they don't take what they see as stupid or unnecessary risks. John McGuinness, one of the most successful riders in the history of the Isle of Man TT, is one of them. 'I think from the outside looking in, it looks like we're taking risks probably 100 per cent of the time when we're on two wheels,' he tells me. 'For me, I take calculated risks – I'd like to think I did. I always leave a little bit in reserve. Looking in, you're like, "Woah!", you know, but I think I have an inner safety barrier that I won't cross.

'You do get a little bit of a buzz and you get a little bit of a warning,' he continues. 'Obviously, that place has claimed a lot of people over the years – over 250 people or whatever – and I think it just gives you a little cheeky warning to say, "Hey, don't push your luck," and you've just got to pull it back a peg or two. It is definitely addictive. But I get more of a rush sometimes when I talk about it and I think about it. You get on the bike and you haven't got time to buzz; things are whizzing past you at, like, 200 miles an hour. Afterwards is more of a buzz – when you cross the line it all runs out of you.'

There seems to be something else going on, on top of the visceral thrill of risking death. 'I'm not sure if adrenaline is exactly the right word,' says wingsuit pilot Alexander Polli, after he's done throwing up in the HPL's bathroom. 'The adrenaline might come during and after the jump potentially, or maybe hours before when I'm hiking up. But if you're talking about five or 10 minutes before, there really isn't a lot of adrenaline at all; it's more of a constant calming.'

'Don't forget that the jump itself is just a small part of what we do,' says Flynn. 'What people don't see in videos is the preparation that goes into each jump. We religiously study maps, weather reports and so on for at least a month before a jump. The end euphoria is not just about the adrenaline rush from doing something crazy. It's an amazing feeling knowing that training, weather and everything came together.'

Adrenaline is not their only motivation.

Dopamine Junkies

You usually hear an avalanche before you see it. If you hear one while descending one of the highest peaks in the Himalayas in the depths of winter, it's supposed to be the last thing you'll ever see. In February 2011, experienced climbers Simone Moro and Denis Urubko, and adventure photographer Cory Richards, became the first people to reach the summit of Gasherbrum II in Pakistan in the winter months.

They were on their way back down when a serac – a huge but fragile chunk of glacial ice – broke off a mountain above with a crack like thunder and landed on the slope above the climbers, triggering an avalanche which picked up speed as it travelled about 1,000 metres downhill. 'We probably turned and managed one step,' remembers 48-year-old Italian Moro when I speak to him and Richards in a plush London hotel six months on. 'It knocked all of us off our feet,' says Richards, whose camera footage of the aftermath of the avalanche is a harrowing watch. 'It rolls you and rolls you for about 150 metres. You just start to see colours as you're spinning – white, light blue, white, dark blue, white, black and then just black, black, black. You realise that you're being pulled under the snow.'

The group were extremely lucky. 'For whatever reason, when I stopped, my face was out of the snow,' remembers Richards. 'My first thought was that I was really mad that I still had to do the descent, and I was upset because Simone and Denis were dead [all three survived]. Then I heard Simone's voice. I was still disoriented, but I felt his hands digging me out to where I could move a little bit, and I started to dig myself.'

Climbing a peak like Gasherbrum II in the winter months is a huge, and some would say unnecessary, risk. It also doesn't come with the adrenaline rush of something like BASE jumping – or at least it shouldn't if everything goes to plan. So what drove the men to do it? 'I do it because I'm in love with the mountains,' says Richards, a young American with blue eyes and ginger hair. 'I love the action and emotions of it all. The point is to do something that has not been done before ... to explore yourself through adventure and do things that have previously been thought of as impossible.'

For the experienced Moro, it was about fulfilling a long-held dream. 'It was not the first time I was attempting to climb a mountain in winter in Pakistan,' he says. 'I had tried it twice before, and once I came within 200 metres of the summit. So when you achieve these dreams that you are postponing and trying for many years, you feel free. But it was not only our common dream, but the dream of an entire climbing community – it's not like a world record, it can't be beaten. It's a sign that even in the third millennium, exploration is not finished. It is a sign that the human never stops exploring.'

The reason humans never stop exploring is the neurotransmitter dopamine. Dopamine produces a sense of satisfaction when we complete a task, whether it's something small like finishing a level on a video game, or something gargantuan like scaling a mountain. 'When you're talking about someone who takes risks to accomplish something,' said neurobiologist Larry Zweifel in a *National Geographic* article, '– climb a mountain, start a company, run for office, become a Navy SEAL – that's driven by motivation, and motivation is driven by the dopamine system. This is what compels humans to move forward.'

One study used fMRI to measure blood flow in the brain as subjects selected from different objects. They found increased activity in the ventral striatum (VS), an area of the brain that is part of the reward system and is involved in releasing dopamine, when they chose unusual objects. 'We think this piece, the VS, adds zing – a reward when we encounter novel things,' one of the researchers, Nathaniel Daw, told *Outside* magazine.

'It's hard,' says TT racer McGuinness. 'It's hard to let go of this drug we all seem to have under our skin.' As a species, our brains are hard-wired by evolution to seek out new things. Rather than adrenaline junkies, some extreme athletes might just be dopamine junkies. But if we're all programmed to seek out new experiences, why is it that some people are so much more enchanted by taking risks than others?

Full Eyes, Clear Hearts, Can't Lose

In the early 1960s, Professor Marvin Zuckerman was running sensory deprivation experiments at the University of Delaware, when he noticed something strange about his volunteers. They were mostly of a certain type – they came carrying motorcycle helmets, and wore their hair long. Why would such free spirits want to sign up for something as ostensibly boring as lying in a darkened, soundproof room for hours at a time?

They'd been drawn by newspaper articles about other sensory deprivation experiments, which reported participants experiencing hallucinations. Zuckerman began to wonder if there was a particular type of person who sought out these kinds of new experiences, and developed a questionnaire to find out. It asks people to agree or disagree with basic statements such as: 'I can't stand watching a movie that I've seen before', or 'I prefer a guide when I am in a place I don't know well'.

From that research he developed the Sensation Seeking Scale, which places people on a spectrum according to how inclined they are to seek out new and potentially dangerous experiences. Subsequent research has found that about 10 per cent of people can be classified as high sensation seekers.

Frank Farley calls these people Type-T thrill-seekers. Now a professor at Temple University in Philadelphia, Farley's interest in risk stems from something that happened when he was eight years old. He was playing in the snow with his friends in Edmonton, Canada, when an elderly neighbour who had been digging his car out of a snowdrift suffered a heart attack. Everyone froze except Farley, who rushed over to try to help. 'I tried to get him into his car so he could lie on the seat rather than the snow,' he remembered in an interview. 'But he died in my arms.' The incident sparked a lifelong passion in Farley, who has spent his career researching why certain people are more likely to step up to the plate in times of need. From interviewing firemen, police officers, paramedics and other people who have risked their own lives to help others, he then went on to develop an interest in whether certain people are more likely to take risks in other situations too.

People with Type-T, or Big-T, personalities are risk-takers – analogous to Zuckerman's high-sensation seekers. 'These people are motivated by risk, uncertainty, novelty, variety,' said Farley. 'They thrive in ambiguous situations. They like intense experiences. They are inner-directed. They believe they can control their fate. Whatever comes up, they believe they can handle it.' The opposite is Type-t, or small-t, personalities – risk-averse people who are motivated by familiarity and certainty.

A Big-T personality can explain involvement in extreme sports, entrepreneurship or creativity in art and science – taking risks in any sphere whether it's mental or physical. Zuckerman defines sensation-seeking behaviour as 'the pursuit of novel and intense experiences without regard for physical, social, legal or financial risk'. The latest versions of his sensation-seeking questionnaire assess people in three categories: their desire for adventure, their disregard for harm, and their impulsivity. High-sensation seekers are more likely to be involved in illegal activities, and more likely to be addicted to drugs. Studies have found similarities between drug addicts in rehab and high-risk sport participants on the Sensation Seeking Scale.

This predilection for risk is partly genetic. It may be down to the way their brains process dopamine – high-sensation seekers may be more stimulated by novelty than your average person because their brains keep producing dopamine for longer. A study at Vanderbilt University, Tennessee, used brain scans to show that high-sensation seekers have fewer dopamine autoreceptors.

Autoreceptors act as an off switch for dopamine. They sit on the outside walls of neurons, but instead of causing the cell to fire, they act as a control mechanism, turning off the flow of neurotransmitters when levels get too high. When the brain of someone with fewer of these autoreceptors is flooded with the dopamine in response to a new experience, they feel it more, and they feel it for longer.

'Think of dopamine like gasoline,' the study's lead author David Zald told *National Geographic*. 'You combine that with a brain equipped with a lesser ability to put on the brakes than normal, and you get people who push limits.'

High-sensation seekers are also more likely to have lower levels of an enzyme called MAO-B (monoamine oxidase B), which breaks down dopamine in the brain. Extreme risk-takers have about a third less MAO-B than the average person, and low levels of it are common to criminals and people with drug or alcohol addiction. Their brains don't break down dopamine as quickly, so it flows around for longer, giving these people more of a high from taking risks. Levels of MAO-B tend to be higher in women, and also increase as we age, which could explain why risk-takers tend to be young and male, and why we tend to mellow as we get older.

Another reason for that is the way the brain's inhibitory system – the prefrontal cortex – develops. It controls our ability to 'put on the brakes' and is the same area that is taxed when we're forcing ourselves not to stop during a long stint on the treadmill.

The reward system in the brain is basic and primal; it governs important behaviours like searching for food in a new environment. As such, it develops much earlier in life – before the inhibitory system has time to catch up when men hit their early twenties – another reason why extreme sports athletes are overwhelmingly young and male, and why adolescent males are generally much more likely to partake in risky behaviour.

Certain people are also better at dealing with fear and anxiety. They have to be. 'I just sweep it to the back of my head,' says McGuinness. 'I've done it for so long now. When you think about what can actually happen ... when it goes wrong, it goes wrong real quick.' Sitting in a tent in the paddock at the Isle of Man TT in 2013, fellow racer Conor Cummins agrees, despite his recent return from a horrific crash on the course that left him with four metal rods in his back and two plates and 16 screws in his left arm. 'There's danger in all walks of life,' he says. 'There's five fucking litres of petrol over there – one nasty spark, we're both burnt to a crisp. If your number's up, your number's up.'

Dr Andy Morgan at Yale Medical School studied two different groups of soldiers going through the US Army's survival school at Fort Bragg in North Carolina. It is hell on earth: 19 days in a mock prisoner-of-war camp complete with guard towers, razor wire and fake graves. The 'prisoners' are subjected to sleep deprivation, semi-starvation and other techniques they might expect to encounter if captured. Morgan compared regular army men with elite special forces soldiers as they went through this experience, and found vastly different levels of a brain chemical called neuropeptide Y.

It works as a natural sedative. Much like the endorphins released during flow, neuropeptide Y helps mitigate the effects of adrenaline. Special forces produced significantly higher levels of neuropeptide Y during survival training, and returned to normal levels quicker than the regular soldiers. This allowed them to remain clear-headed when under extreme stress and experiencing fear – a vitally important ability when the wrong decision could mean death or capture.

The US Navy have a unique and rather brutal way of working out which of their new recruits will be best suited to risky underwater missions. They quite literally throw them in at the deep end. At the Navy Diving and Salvage Training Center in Florida, they bind the feet of young sailors and tie their hands behind their backs. Then they chuck them in an Olympic-sized pool with the challenge of staying afloat. A lot of them black out and have to be pulled out by divers. 'The more someone struggles,' Morgan told *Newsweek*, 'the harder it is to get air and the more tired they get. You just have to inhibit the powerful, incredible instinct to breathe, and your anxiety and alarm.'

Morgan found a correlation between performances on this test and the levels of neuropeptide Y in the brain. The more neuropeptide Y the sailors had, the quicker the adrenaline was broken down, and the faster they were able to regain control and calm down their breathing. Underwater divers in another stressful situation also had different brain chemistry – they released higher amounts of DHEA, a natural steroid which counteracts the effects of the stress hormone cortisol.

Brain chemistry can predict whether you'll seek out high-risk activities, and how well you'll cope with the fear and anxiety that they create. Morgan also thinks he's found a quick way of determining who will perform the best under pressure. He measured the heartbeats of soldiers waiting to head into close-quarters combat training – a simulated battle with fake ammunition that really hurts. The soldiers who had more metronomic heartbeats performed better. Their heartbeat was more regular, and the gaps between beats didn't vary as much as it does in most people – possibly because their brainstem, which controls heartbeat, has a higher concentration of neuropeptide Y-releasing cells. Perhaps a list of players with more metronomic heart rates could prove useful for a manager deciding who should take penalties in a vital shoot-out. The calmer the heart, the calmer the mind.

Don't Fear The Reaper

There's remote, and then there's Sam Ford Fjord on the north-east coast of Baffin Island, the largest of Canada's snow-covered satellites and the fifth largest island in the world. It's two and a half times the size of Great Britain, but has a population of just 11,000. If you want to get around, your options are dog sleds or snowmobiles.

In April 2010, a group of 20 elite BASE jumpers took the second option – seven hours of it – when they spent a month on the island honing their skills on some of the biggest cliff faces on the planet. They pitched up at the foot of Kigut Peak, a 1,000-metre cliff face supposedly named after the Inuit word for teeth. They built snow walls, igloo-style, to protect their tents from the fierce winds, and spent their days (weather permitting) climbing and jumping and climbing again.

Ted Davenport was one of the group, and he had something even more spectacular in mind: he wanted to emulate James Bond. *The Spy Who Loved Me* opens with a scene set in Austria, but actually shot on Baffin Island's Mount Asgard, in which Roger Moore's Bond flees from some assailants on skis, and ends up skiing straight off the side of a mountain. The sequence, ably performed by stuntman Rick Sylvester, ends with Bond pulling a cord to reveal a Union Jack parachute.

Davenport hails from Aspen, Colorado, and comes from a family of professional skiers. He didn't have quite the same level of patriotism in mind, but he did do something equally spectacular. After a few days of scouting for locations, he found an ideal spot for skiing: a natural bowl of snow with one outlet – a frozen waterfall. Davenport skied off the edge of the waterfall – a 2,000-foot drop to the fjord below. In doing so he became the first person to 'ski-BASE' on Baffin Island since 007.

'Every time I step off the edge I'm scared,' he says in a short online documentary. 'Every single time. When it gets to the point that you're not scared you probably shouldn't jump any more. It's that fear that keeps you sharp, keeps you focused, keeps you alive. It's knowing that if I make a mistake, if I do something wrong, this is what can happen.'

But despite that, it seems that Davenport's brain may process fear entirely differently from someone less daring. In 2009, he went into UCLA's fMRI scanner to have his brain activity measured for an article in *Outside* magazine. He played a computer game called the Balloon Analogue Risk Task. In this task, the participant sees a cartoon balloon which inflates as they press a button. The more it inflates, the more points they win, but it will randomly pop at some point and, if it does, they'll lose everything. There's another button that allows the participant to cash out and take what they have before the balloon bursts, like taking the money on *Who Wants to Be a Millionaire?*

Most people play the task quite safe and, when a balloon bursts, the fMRI shows activity in their amygdala, the seat of fear and the fight, flight, freeze response. But, as we've seen in this chapter, the brains of people who risk their lives for a living behave quite differently.

When his balloon has burst, Davenport's amygdala shows up blank. But his ventral striatum – the area of the brain associated with pleasure and the 'zing' of dopamine – lights up like a Christmas tree. Davenport's brain treats loss completely differently. Despite what he says, he seems to have no fear of it.

CHAPTER THIRTEEN

IN SEARCH OF SPORTING IQ

Vincent Kompany speaks five languages and has a master's degree from Manchester Business School. He is the captain of Manchester City and Belgium, and one of football's most articulate interviewees, as I found out when I spoke to him for *Sport* in October 2015. When he started his career, the central defender's play was flashy, with superfluous tricks and stepovers, but as he got older he learnt to strip those aspects out of his game. 'It wouldn't have been a great sign of intelligence on my part if I was still doing tricks as a defender,' he tells me. 'What I know and what I've realised is that actually to be the best defender I need to do something else, so what you do is kind of evolve and understand, "OK, this is what I need to do." And I think players like Cristiano Ronaldo are a good example, you know?'

The Portuguese forward wasn't always the goalscoring machine he is now. When he first signed for Manchester United, Ronaldo was a tricky yet frustrating winger; clearly talented, but not always capable of making the right decision. 'You see Cristiano Ronaldo for Man United, and you see Cristiano Ronaldo now, and some people will always say that they prefer the Ronaldo that was doing the tricks and stuff, but in reality the best Ronaldo ever for his team is the Ronaldo that you see in the last two or three years,' says Kompany. 'That is intelligence.'

'For that he needs to decide that he's going to be in certain positions, getting the ball at certain times, managing his body in a certain way and stripping out certain things that weren't giving him those statistics.' Kompany doesn't think there's a link between intelligence on the pitch and off it. 'You see the most surprising people turning out to be extremely intelligent on the pitch. For me, it's two different types of intelligence.'

The Wonderlic test is a search for intelligence. It's a small part of the unique spectacle of the NFL Scouting Combine. Every March, a couple of months before the draft where the teams pick which college players they want to add to their ranks, all those hopefuls undergo a battery of tests. NFL commentator Neil Reynolds calls it 'a head-spinning combination of a cattle market and a speed-dating session'.

Every aspect of a player's physique is measured and scrutinised, from the size of their calves to their body fat percentage, as well as blood pressure and organ function. The Combine is a place for extraordinary feats of athleticism, the likes of which you're unlikely to see outside of the Olympics. Players jump seemingly impossible distances from standing positions, run passing drills like pros, and set 40-yard dash times that would see them on the verge of medals in an elite athletics competition.

They also undergo a mental assessment. The Wonderlic test consists of 50 questions, and players are given 12 minutes to answer as many as they can. It's a boiled-down version of an IQ test, measuring the prospective NFL players' ability to think and reason quickly and accurately. A typical question is: *A boy is 17 years old and his sister is twice as old. When the boy is 23 years old, what will be the age of his sister?*

The reasoning behind the Wonderlic test is that for players who have to make decisions – in American football that's usually the quarterback – it's important to have an agile mind as well as a good throwing arm. There are few lengths to which scouts at elite level won't go to try to get an edge on their opponents. One company, Achievement Metrics, even promises to analyse everything a player has said in public to assess the likelihood that they will 'have trouble following team rules', 'miss games because of off-field behaviour' or even 'be arrested while under contract'.

Since the 1970s, NFL scouts have been using the Wonderlic test on the assumption that maths and reasoning skills equate to a better ability to memorise hundreds of plays and defensive formations, and pick the right pass under pressure. According to *ESPN* magazine, the unofficial average score for a quarterback on the Wonderlic test is 24, compared to 16 for running backs, 29 for computer programmers and 15 for janitors. But does it actually make a difference? Some of the best quarterbacks in the sport's history did not excel on the test (Dan Marino scored 15), while others who scored highly went on to struggle in the NFL.

A study by economists David Berri and Rob Simmons in 2009 looked at whether Wonderlic scores had any bearing on success as a quarterback. They found that IQ, as measured by the test, was as important as height or 40-yard dash time in determining whether a quarterback got selected in the draft, but had no value when predicting their actual performance in the NFL. In fact, there was a slight negative correlation between Wonderlic scores and quarterback performance in the first year of players' careers. It seems that sporting intelligence is not quite the same as intelligence in other fields, and indeed NFL coaches are starting to put less weight on Wonderlic scores when drafting players, especially as evidence suggests that practice can improve performance on the test dramatically. Former Cincinnati quarterback Akili Smith's score improved from 12 the first time he took it to 37 the second time around.

In Parts One and Two, we looked at sport-specific aspects of sporting intelligence such as anticipation and high-speed decision-making, and how they can be trained. But what if we want to identify people whose brains are primed for sporting success before they've been trained? If the Wonderlic test doesn't predict sporting success, is there a general measure of 'sporting IQ' that can?

Neural Giants

Most people don't grow up with a skeleton track in their back garden or anywhere nearby, but a gold medal is a gold medal, so for years national Olympic associations have implemented talent identification programmes for some of the more niche sports, particularly in the Winter Olympics, looking for people who might have the skills or the physique to become elite athletes in a completely new field. Olympic skeleton champion Lizzy Yarnold was originally a heptathlete, who was recruited for a new sport because of her strength, speed and co-ordination.

Certain people have innate physical advantages when it comes to sport that have very little to do with how much they've practised. There's a great stat from David Epstein's *The Sports Gene* which points out that if you're an American male between the ages of 18 and 40 and you're over seven feet tall, there's a 17 per cent chance that you're a *current* NBA player.

The intangible sporting IQ is the brain's equivalent of these physical gifts, and it could become a highly prized asset as scouts continue to try to gain an advantage over their opponents by recruiting athletes earlier, and as they try to identify those with the greatest potential for improvement not just in the body but in the mind.

General sporting intelligence is a slippery concept. It is more than highly trained anticipation and recognition-primed decision-making. If you had to identify someone likely to excel across a range of sports from just their mental abilities, working memory capacity would be one of the most telling metrics. Working memory is a measure of how much information someone can hold in their head. It has been linked to reading comprehension, problem-solving and IQ, but it applies equally to sport. The more information you can hold in your head at once, the less prone you are to distractions, and the quicker and better you can make decisions.

One study of ice hockey players found that those with a low working memory capacity failed to adjust their tactical decisions to the game situation, and instead just blindly followed instructions from their coaches, even when they weren't appropriate. Players with a higher working memory capacity were better at adjusting their tactical decision-making to the situation in the game, in this case a fictional scenario created for the study.

When it comes to performance, working memory is just as important as how much someone knows, or how much experience they have. In 2002, David Hambrick and colleagues at Michigan State University tested a group of people on their overall baseball knowledge and interest with a series of questionnaires, and their working memory with a couple of computer tasks.

Finally, the participants were asked to listen to recordings of fictional baseball games, and tested on their ability to remember details from the games, such as the score, the number of outs, or the batting averages of particular players. The results revealed that the people who knew more about baseball were better at recalling information from the games – unsurprising given what we know about chunking. But working memory capacity was also strongly linked to success, at both high and low levels of baseball knowledge.

Another study with piano players found similar results. A group of 57 pianists with lifetime practice hours ranging from between 260 to 31,000 had their working memory capacity tested before being given a piece of music they had never seen before to sight read. Practice was obviously an important predictor of success – it accounted for about half of the difference in their sight-reading performance. But it wasn't the only predictor. Working memory capacity had an effect on their performance too, above and beyond their level of experience. It's not just about how many hours you've put in; underlying mental faculties such as working memory can also impact on performance.

When the concept of working memory was first described in the 1970s, people set about trying to expand their capacity. Steve Faloon, a college student with 'average intelligence' and 'average memory abilities', spent an hour a day, between three and five days a week for a year, training his ability to remember numbers. Random digits were read out to him at a rate of one per second, and then he was asked to recall the sequence. Over the course of 230 hours of training, Faloon was able to increase the number of digits he could accurately recall from seven to 79 – seemingly, an amazing expansion of his working memory capacity.

However, this has more to do with chunking than an actual increase in working memory capacity. In the same way that expert athletes develop processing strategies to help them read the action and remember it better than non-experts, Faloon simply developed a mnemonic to help him remember the digits better. His working memory capacity hadn't improved, as neatly demonstrated by this: although he could recall almost 80 numbers in a row, he could only manage to remember six random letters at a time.

Working memory capacity can't be trained, and it does have an impact on sporting performance. These neural giants may not be quite as easy for scouts to spot as seven-foot-tall basketball players, but they could well be worth finding.

Fluent Football

Fortunately, for any aspiring athletes who can't remember a phone number, working memory capacity is not the only mental faculty that has been linked to sporting success. Athletes also perform better on measures of processing speed, attention and executive function.

Executive function is an umbrella term encompassing a wide range of mental abilities including problem-solving, planning, inhibition, decision-making, and the ability to update information being held in working memory (although not working memory capacity itself). It correlates closely with success in many walks of life, including sport.

In one study of executive function, Laura Chaddock at the University of Illinois asked college students to walk in front of traffic. Well, virtual traffic anyway – a simulated city scene comprised of three screens arranged in a U-shape, and a synchronised treadmill, like a souped-up version of arcade game *Frogger*.

She compared 16 student athletes across a range of sports with 16 equally smart and similarly aged non-athletes on their ability to safely walk (they weren't allowed to run) across this virtual road, which had cars going by at 40 to 50 miles per hour. The athletes were significantly better.

One study of Swedish footballers used a 'design fluency' test as part of a series of measures of executive function. In the design fluency test, the players were presented with a series of squares filled with dots, and were given a pen and 60 seconds to find as many different ways of joining the dots as possible, without repeating any.

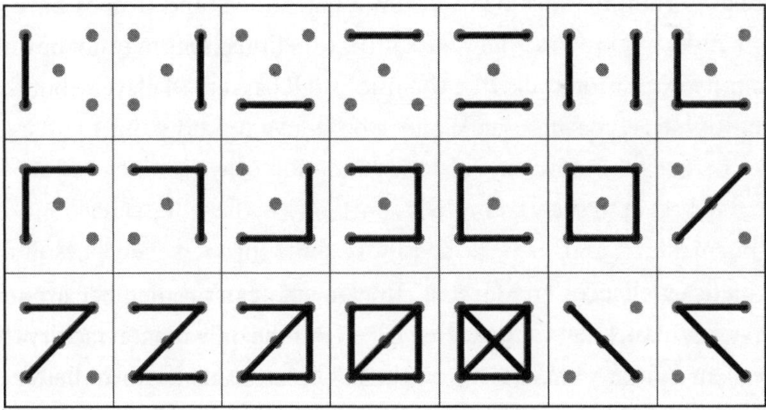

To do this well, they needed to use a number of executive functions: planning a systematic strategy, inhibition to avoid repeating previous responses and scanning for new solutions to the task.

The researchers tested 57 players from the top two professional divisions in Swedish football on this and other tests, and found that the players had significantly better executive functions than a group of non-players. The players in the top division, the Allsvenskan, were also better than the players from the league below.

Over the following two seasons, the researchers kept track of the 57 players they had tested, to look for stronger evidence of a link between executive function and on-pitch success. They found a clear link between scores on the design fluency test and the number of goals and assists over the following two seasons, even after controlling for age and position.

'In ball-sports like soccer there are large amounts of information for the players to consider in every new moment,' they write. 'The successful player must constantly assess the situation, compare it to past experiences, create new possibilities, make quick decisions to action, but also quickly inhibit planned decisions. Thus, several core-features of executive functions such as planning, sustained and divided attention, suppression of previous responses, and working memory capacity are important for a team player in soccer.'

Unlike working memory, executive functions *can* be trained, with cognitive training tools like the ones we looked at in Part Two. The question that coaches and scouts would love to know the answer to is whether the improved executive function of elite athletes is what enabled them to succeed in their sport, or whether they started out at a normal level and then trained those skills through their pursuit of athletic excellence. Jan Mayer at Hoffenheim has seen an improvement in performances on the gruelling DT-Wiener test of executive function year on year as players train on the pitch, but in truth it's probably a bit of both.

As with muscle strength or aerobic capacity, people start at different levels and improve at different rates. As sport pushes the boundaries ever further, teams and scouts in search of athletes with potential will have to tap into why.

Genetic Scouting

This book contains about 100,000 words, which is about half a million characters, including spaces. Imagine (or buy) 6,000 copies and you get 3 billion characters – the number of letters in the human genome. Those letters are formed by four amino acids – adenine, cytosine, guanine and thymine – which arrange themselves into pairs along the rungs of the twisted rope ladder that is a DNA molecule.

Taken together, these letters are the blueprint for everything that makes you. The sequence of letters is arranged across 23 pairs of chromosomes, but can also be broken down into smaller parts, called genes, each of which contains the recipe for a particular structure or protein in your body. Almost every cell, every hair, every drop of blood contains a copy of every gene – there are between 20,000 and 25,000 different genes – and they interact in intricate ways to code for the remarkable complexity of the human body.

Sports teams have already started using genetics to profile their players and assess them for risk of injury. A British company called DNAFit has worked with some Premier League football teams, using genetic markers to help identify areas in which training programmes can be targeted towards individual players' genetic make-up.

'There's not going to be a single gene that determines success or failure,' DNAFit's chief scientific officer Dr Keith Grimaldi told the *Daily Mail*. 'There's no "Lionel Messi gene", but we can help people to work with the genetics they have.' Grimaldi thinks the use of genetics in sport will only grow in future. 'I will be very surprised if, over the next several years, it does not become absolutely routine,' he said. 'It should be. We're not promising magic but we're just hoping to reduce the risk. It's like wearing a seat belt or looking both ways before you cross the road.'

He was less enthusiastic about the potential use of genetic testing for scouting purposes. 'It would be no different to all the other techniques that are used to determine which sport, such as arm or leg length;

things that are already visible in children. Most of the information in selecting a sport or spotting talent is there for us to see with a stopwatch or tape measure,' he said.

While that's true of physical characteristics, it is not the case for mental factors such as working memory or executive function. Surely it won't be too long before teams and coaches start looking at neural genetics too, perhaps to assess potential when recruiting players. Anything to get an edge.

Different people have different versions of particular genes – one variant might code for a particular hair colour, for example – although often it's the interplay between different genes and our environment that determines how we end up. To get around this problem and prise apart nature and nurture, genetics researchers spend a lot of time looking for twins. Identical twins share the same set of genes, while non-identical twins don't. Therefore, by comparing large groups of identical and non-identical twins on a particular trait, researchers can assess to what extent it is determined by genes. Because twins tend to share an environment, if identical twins are considerably more similar in a particular facet than non-identical twins, then it means genes have an important role to play.

Working memory researchers using this strategy compared hundreds of pairs of identical and non-identical twins in Japan. Genetics accounted for two-thirds of the difference in their spatial working memory abilities.

One version of a gene called COMT has been linked with improved performance in working memory tasks, and reduced activity in the prefrontal cortex during those tasks. The neurotransmitter dopamine plays a key role in working memory in this area of the brain, and it's thought that the COMT gene may play a role in how quickly it gets broken down, although there are conflicting results.

Other genes have been identified that are linked to processing speed and the brain's ability to control and switch focus between tasks. One twin study estimated that individual differences in executive function are almost entirely genetic.

So although the brain is plastic, and can be shaped by its environment, genes do play a role in its basic biology and can have a knock-on effect on working memory, executive function and, by extension, sporting intelligence. We already know that people with certain genes are better suited physically to certain sports, and the same could be true for the brain and sporting IQ.

Sometimes, even just a one-letter difference in the 3 billion character sequence of DNA can have a profound impact on the body, or on the brain. Certain people improve their aerobic capacity much more rapidly with training than others, and this difference in trainability can be at least partly explained by genetics.

Dr Claude Bouchard tested identical twins and pairs of brothers in three studies to see how their VO_2 max (how much oxygen the body can consume while exercising – how fit they are, basically) changed when they went through identical training plans. The range of responses to training was between six and nine times larger for brothers than for identical twins, and eventually, through the HERITAGE family study, Bouchard identified 21 gene variants that predict how an individual's aerobic capacity – their fitness level – will respond to training.

The brain's own trainability – its plasticity – could also have a genetic component, and it's one that's determined by just a one-letter swap in one of the base pairs that make up DNA. This swap results in a slightly different amino acid being made. Amino acids are the building blocks of proteins, so this switch results in some people having a slightly different version of the protein called brain-derived neurotrophic factor (BDNF). You might remember BDNF from chapter three. It boosts the growth of new connections in the brain, may trigger critical periods, and also explains the improvement in learning and memory we get when we exercise. It is the brain's natural growth hormone. The gene on the 11th chromosome which contains the blueprint for BDNF is called the BDNF gene, and there are two different types.

About 65 per cent of people have the Val66Val version of the gene, while about 35 per cent have the Val66Met version. The latter version makes a type of BDNF that is a slightly different shape from the 'normal' type, which the majority of people have. It doesn't get distributed around neurons quite as easily, and so when they fire, about 30 per cent less BDNF is released. The Val66Met version of the gene has been associated with abnormal cortical development, memory impairments and reduced activity in the medial temporal cortex. It has also been linked to lower levels of neural plasticity.

One study used TMS (transcranial magnetic stimulation) to measure the brain activity of people while they practised simple motor tasks such as tapping keyboard keys as quickly as possible. They found a change in the level of electrical impulses being sent from the brain to the muscles, but only in the participants who had the more common Val66Val version of the BDNF gene. The brains of people with this version of the gene may be more able to change with experience; they are more trainable.

Born To Run

Becoming an elite athlete is not an easy process. Even with some of the potential shortcuts we've looked at, it still takes dedication and hours upon hours of hard work on the training field. One of the biggest things that differentiates athletes and non-athletes is their propensity to put the effort in – to sacrifice now in the pursuit of a future goal. That's true regardless of any genetic advantages they might have.

Even Finnish cross-country skier Eero Mantyranta, whose mutated EPOR gene gave him the ability to carry 50 per cent extra oxygen in his blood, still had to put in the effort to unlock his gift and win seven Winter Olympic medals.

It takes thousands of hours to become an expert. Some of the training tools we looked at in Part Two could help shorten that process, but there may be a way of differentiating people before they get to that stage. Neuroscience could help predict which young athletes have the determination and dedication to reach the top of their sport before they've even stepped on to a training pitch or picked up a bat.

The Finns have a concept which doesn't neatly fit a single English word in translation – something that speaks to their nation's character, up there in the cold on the fringes of Russia. It's called *sisu*, and it means something like bravery, or determination – perseverance. Mantyranta had it. So did Mika Hakkinen, who won two Formula 1 world titles, battling against the dominance of Ferrari and Michael Schumacher. 'In English, *sisu* means courage,' he has said.

Angela Lee Duckworth might call it grit. 'Grit is passion and perseverance for very long-term goals,' she said in a TED talk. 'Grit is having stamina. Grit is sticking with your future, day in, day out, not just for the week, not just for the month, but for years, and working really hard to make that future a reality. Grit is living life like it's a marathon, not a sprint.'

Duckworth, a Harvard and Oxford graduate, was working as a management consultant but had an abrupt career change at the age of 27. 'I left a very demanding job for a job that was even more demanding: teaching,' she said. 'I went to teach seventh graders in the New York City public schools. And like any teacher, I made quizzes and tests. I gave out homework assignments. When the work came back, I calculated grades. What struck me was that IQ was not the only difference between my best and worst students.'

She has studied military cadets, spelling bee contestants, salespeople and teachers. 'In all those very different contexts, one characteristic emerged as a significant predictor of success,' she said. 'And it wasn't social intelligence. It wasn't good looks, or physical health, and it wasn't IQ. It was grit.'

If talent is a result of deliberate practice, then grit is the driving force behind practice. It's the mental strength to get out of bed early in the morning to go swimming, to practise three hours a day after school, to stay behind after training to work on free kicks. 'I'd bet that there isn't a single highly successful person who hasn't depended on grit,' Duckworth told ESPN. 'Nobody is talented enough to not have to work hard, and that's what grit allows you to do. It lets you take advantage of your potential. In order to become a professional athlete, you need a certain kind of obsessiveness. You've got to devote your life to the development of this very narrow expertise. It shouldn't be surprising that this takes lots of grit.'

Measurement of grit takes the form of a simple eight- or 12-item questionnaire with statements such as 'Setbacks don't discourage me', and then five options to choose from ranging from 'very much like me' to 'not like me at all'.

You get assigned points, from one to five, for each question depending on your responses, add them up like you're doing a quiz in a 1990s pop music magazine, and then divide by the number of questions and that's your grit score out of five. Mine is 2.63, according to one version of the test, which I think makes it slightly miraculous that I've made it this far into writing the book without fleeing to Mexico or something.

It's not a particularly sophisticated measurement, but it is a powerful one. In one study, Duckworth tested contestants at the National Spelling Bee – an American concept almost wholly alien on these shores, in which children are pitted against each other on their ability to spell arcane words. In 2006, the year Duckworth was testing, the competition was won by a 13-year-old girl who successfully spelled the word 'ursprache' from the definition, 'a hypothetically reconstructed parent language'. Me neither.

Working with K. Anders Ericsson and others, Duckworth tested the 273 spellers on their 'grittiness' with an eight-point questionnaire, and also asked them how much time they spent engaged in various revision activities, including looking at flashcards and being quizzed on their spelling. She found that the best spellers had put in the most deliberate practice; they'd spent the most time doing the boring bits of learning, looking at flashcards rather than being quizzed, for example.

They were also, without question, the grittiest, scoring higher on the scale. Grit leads to deliberate practice leads to success. So maybe instead of searching for sporting IQ or the million-dollar brain, scouts need to find the young athletes with the grit and determination to put the hours in, even if they're not very good at first.

But where does this quality come from? Grit is not linked to intelligence or talent. The propensity to get up and go is one aspect of grit, and it could be partly genetic. A number of twin studies, including one that used accelerometers to directly measure movement, have found that identical twins are more likely to have similar activity levels than non-identical twins – a sure-fire sign that there is some genetic basis to the trait. One study of more than 37,000 pairs of twins from seven different countries found that genetics could account for between half and three-quarters of the variation in the amount of exercise they did – way more than any environmental factors.

Theodore Garland discovered something similar when he bred mice that were born to run. Garland, a physiologist at UC Riverside in California, separated a group of average mice into two groups based on how long they chose to run on a wheel each night. He bred the high runners together and the low runners together, over a number of generations. By the 16th generation, the high running group were voluntarily running seven miles a night, while the other group ran four miles a night.

This difference is also thought to be due to the dopamine system – the brain's reward mechanism. In the last chapter, we saw how dopamine may be the reason why some people are more inclined to take risks, and it could also explain why some are more inclined to exert themselves physically as well.

Like all neurotransmitters, dopamine works by binding itself to receptors on the outside of neurons, which opens channels that eventually cause the neuron to fire an electrical impulse. It's like a key in a lock. The dopamine receptors – the keyholes – are made inside the neuron and then get transported to the outside surfaces to do their job.

Joint research published last year by the University of Aberdeen and the Chinese Academy of Sciences found a gene, called SLC35D3, which affects how these dopamine receptors are transported. They nicknamed it 'the couch potato gene' because mice with this gene walk around only a third as much as other mice, and move more slowly. In mice with this gene, the receptors are made as normal, but end up getting stuck inside the cells, leaving the neurons with fewer dopamine receptors – fewer locks and doors to be opened. It's harder to get them to fire. The brains of mice with this gene found the release of dopamine that accompanies reward less stimulating, so they were less inclined to seek it out.

Other genetic mutations affecting dopamine receptors have been associated with *higher* levels of physical activity, including the 7R variant of the DRD4 gene. People with these genes have more dopamine receptors, so it's easier to get their neurons to fire. As a result, they do more. They're grittier.

When people talk about innate talent, perhaps they should be talking about innate drive, innate grit, or innate dopamine sensitivity. But very little in the brain is fixed at birth. 'Science says grit comes from both nature and nurture,' Duckworth told the *Washington Post*. 'There was a belief for a long time that once someone's character is set, it never changes. There's this saying: "Give me the child; I'll show you the man." But empirical data shows the contrary: people do change in their traits and that continues all across the life course. Earlier in life, in childhood and adolescence, change is more dramatic. But people in their fifties still evolve.'

As with almost everything in the plastic brain, you can override your genetics if you believe you can; and it's that belief in your ability to change which could be the most crucial component of grit. Your willingness to work hard, your grit, is still an important predictor of sporting success no matter how well you train your brain, but the overarching lesson from psychology and neuroscience is that it's in your own hands. Adopt the right mindset, and you can do anything.

Learning From Mistakes

When Vincent Kompany first started playing football, he wasn't very good. He learnt to play on the streets, at the foot of the tower blocks of his home in northern Brussels, and joined the youth set-up at local club Anderlecht at the age of six. But his first goal was an own goal. He made himself better through sheer force of will. Through grit. 'I was incredibly stubborn and I just wanted to learn,' he tells me. Kompany was quick and strong, but not as good on the ball as his peers.

'Very early on people were telling me: "This is what you're good at", because I was already strong and probably a bit taller than the other kids, so they said, "Do this, do that." I never really accepted it. I wanted to do what the smaller kids were doing; I wanted to be as technical and as gifted as they were. They had it naturally but with hard work I eventually developed a really good technique and started becoming a very complete footballer. I kept always thinking, what someone else can do, I can do.'

Kompany has what psychologist Carol Dweck has called a 'growth mindset'. According to Dweck, people with a growth mindset believe that ability comes from hard work and dedication; that 'talent' is just a baseline and that they can improve over time. A 'fixed mindset' is the opposite – the belief that talent or intelligence are fixed; you get your lot and there's nothing you can do about it, regardless of how much effort you put in. People with a growth mindset are much more likely to be gritty. They'll put in the hours because, like Kompany, they believe that they can improve.

Fostering a growth mindset has become a hot topic in coaching and education. Advice for doing so includes praising effort over ability. Rather than gushing at talent, we should reward graft to help encourage the idea that people are in command of their own destiny.

I asked Kompany where he thought his determination, his grit, his growth mindset came from. He cites both his parents – his father from Congo, his mother French-Belgian – as a huge influence. 'My dad used to play football in Africa, so he was playing for nothing but he was playing in front of stadiums filled with 60, 70, 80,000 people sometimes. He came [to Europe] as a political refugee, and he's had a lot of ups and downs in his life. He still talks about Congo as being a very great country where he grew up, but obviously he was forced by the regime at the time to leave the country, fearing for his life. When he came here he was studying; he became a taxi driver. All these things are kind of embedded in the family, whichever way we go, whatever we achieve.'

Overcoming adversity is a common narrative thread in the history of many sports stars – from playing football in the street, to escaping a life of crime or destitution. Early childhood trauma can make people grittier, more adaptable and better at dealing with stressful situations. There's some evidence that this ability could even be passed down to children; if parents have been through a lot, their offspring may inherit that adaptability.

The brains of people with a growth mindset react to setbacks differently. The brain has two immediate responses to a mistake. The first, called error-related negativity (ERN), is an involuntary response that happens about 50 milliseconds after we make a mistake and is thought to originate in the anterior cingulate cortex, an area of the brain that monitors risk and reward. Between 100 and 500 milliseconds after a mistake comes a second signal, error positivity (Pe), which is associated with our awareness of the error.

The larger the ERN and Pe signals, the better people learn from their mistakes. There's a bigger initial response to the error, and they're paying more attention to it. In 2010, Jason Moser conducted an EEG experiment at Michigan State University. He wanted to see whether there was a difference in these responses depending on mindset. He gave undergraduates a mindset questionnaire, which is similar in set-up to Duckworth's grit test, and asks to what extent people agree with statements such as: 'You have a certain amount of intelligence and cannot do much to change it.'

He divided the students into two groups based on their responses: a fixed mindset group and a growth mindset group. Then, he hooked them up to an EEG and gave them a computer-based task. They looked at five-letter sequences such as BBBBB or BBGBB and had to identify the middle letter each time. Occasionally, they would get it wrong, and Moser examined their brain waves when they made these mistakes. The initial reaction in both groups was the same: they showed a large ERN signal – 'the brain sits up and pays attention when things go wrong,' is how Matthew Syed puts it in *Black Box Thinking*.

But the Pe signal was vastly different. The growth mindset group showed a much higher neural response to a mistake – three times larger than those in the fixed mindset group. The size of the Pe signal was also directly correlated with the degree to which people's performances improved after their mistakes.

The brains of people with a growth mindset treat failure differently, and thus they respond to it in a more constructive manner, and learn from it. Regardless of any innate sporting intelligence or physical talent, athletes with a growth mindset believe they can get better through hard work and dedication. Although, as we've seen in this chapter, some people's brains may be innately less trainable, or less suited to certain sports, it doesn't mean those obstacles can't be overcome. Adopting a growth mindset creates grit, and grit leads to success.

'We don't like defeat,' says Kompany. 'And if we do lose, then we always come back somehow trying to see if we can actually do better. It's a mindset in the whole family.'

CHAPTER FOURTEEN

OUTCASTS AND OPPORTUNITIES

Aaron Cook used to be a prodigy. Now he is an outcast. At 17, he went to the 2008 Beijing Olympic Games to represent Great Britain in taekwondo – a frenetic martial art with an emphasis on fast and accurate kicking. Now, though, the three-time European champion doesn't compete for his country of birth. At the Rio Olympics and beyond, Cook will fight for Moldova.

Seven weeks before the 2011 World Championships, GB Taekwondo, which runs the sport's world-class performance programme in the UK, pulled Cook's coach. His replacement was someone Cook had never worked with before, and the fighter's results deteriorated. He suffered a shock first-round defeat.

After that, Cook decided to quit the programme, turning his back on up to £100,000 a year of funding to find and finance his own coaching instead. His results improved almost immediately under his new coaching regime, but he believes that his decision to quit the formal set-up was held against him the following year. In the run-up to the 2012 Olympics in London, Cook was world number one and had won nine of his previous 12 tournaments. But he was not selected for the Games.

Instead, GB Taekwondo chose Lutalo Muhammad, who was 58 places below Cook in the world rankings at the time. Despite multiple appeals, and investigations by the British Olympic Association and the World Taekwondo Federation, the decision eventually stuck, and Cook was denied the chance to compete at his home Olympics.

He was heartbroken, and felt he had been the victim of a decision motivated by non-sporting considerations. Under the circumstances, Cook decided that, with the short career open to him at the highest level, he had no other choice but to change nationality. 'Moldova approached me first,' he said of his switch, after his citizenship was reportedly funded by the billionaire president of the Eastern European country's taekwondo federation. 'They could make everything happen very fast and very easy. It was the perfect situation. I have found it very easy to switch. It is exactly the same mat, the same arena. It is just that I have different letters on the back of my suit.'

So, instead of preparing for Rio at the recently refurbished Taekwondo Academy in Manchester, Cook has been training alone in a low-slung brick unit on an industrial estate on the outskirts of the city, still working with one of the coaches who helped him turn his form around after he left the formal set-up.

He has been getting ready in a very different way from his former colleagues too. Cook has been training his brain.

I get a Manchester welcome when I pay a visit to the brain gym – the first noise I hear is rain pinging off the corrugated metal roof of the long, low unit, which sits among old factories and converted or vacant warehouses in Ashton-under-Lyne, Greater Manchester. There's a sign above the door which reads: 'Mick Clegg – Seed of Speed'. Inside, it looks like an ordinary, if untidy, gym, with the usual array of weights and racks, and gym mats stacked in haphazard piles. To the right, there's a ping-pong table where Aaron Cook – tall and powerful, with dark hair and a few days of stubble – is showing off an impressive range of table-tennis shots. To the left, a young footballer called Pierre sits on a low wooden bench, tapping away at an iPad. In front of him, there's a square area of padded flooring that's been roped off, a bit like a boxing ring, with a flat-screen television on one side, facing inwards. All around, footballs hang from ropes on the low ceiling.

At the far end, there's a small room that serves as an office, among other things. A sign on the lintel says 'The Cave', and there are two posters on the flimsy wooden door – one of a cheetah, and the other of a peregrine falcon in flight. Mick Clegg calls me in. He's reclining in an armchair, wearing slippers and wrapped in a thick blanket against the November chill. I feel like I've been summoned for an audience with the leader of a medieval gang. Clegg is in his fifties, but looks much younger, and has piercing blue eyes and the brusque yet friendly manner that comes from years of trying to keep young athletes in line.

Clegg's journey into brain training started when he worked at Manchester United between 2000 and 2011, as a power development coach at the club's training ground, Carrington. Two of his sons played for the club, although only one – Michael – made a first-team appearance. His office is lined with signed shirts and pictures of former United players.

When Clegg joined the club, Sir Alex Ferguson's team had just won the treble – Premier League, Champions League and FA Cup – and initially his work was centred around building speed and strength in the gym, which he tried to do by tailoring exercises to each individual player's needs. He worked with the likes of Roy Keane and Ruud van Nistelrooy, right the way through to Wayne Rooney and Cristiano Ronaldo, who transformed from a lightweight winger to a muscular forward during his time at the club, partly with Clegg's help.

Although Clegg started out with weight machines and boxing routines in Carrington's vast gym, his work slowly morphed into something different. 'Most players don't look at being stronger, they look at being faster,' he says. 'Being stronger doesn't necessarily give you much more ammunition, but speed does. How do you develop power, with speed being the main ingredient? Of course it all comes from the brain. You realise, when you start training elite sportspeople, that it's the brain that is really important, because it's the brain that controls everything. So you look at all the ways of training that.

'A third of what the brain is used for is vision,' he tells me, indicating the two posters on his office door – the cheetah and the peregrine falcon. The cheetah is the fastest animal on land, capable of running at speeds of up to 70mph, while the peregrine falcon is the fastest creature on earth. It can reach 220mph in a dive.

'Why are they so fast?' asks Clegg, gesticulating wildly. 'Is it because he flaps his wings so quick, or because he pounds his feet into the floor so quick? No. It's actually about vision.'

The reason athletes are able to react at seemingly superhuman speeds is because they have trained their visual abilities – their sport-specific skills of anticipation and pattern recognition. The best athletes know where to look to get the information they need. 'What we need to do as athletes,' says Clegg, 'is realise that our vision is what is going to give us the opportunity to get to that ball, to be able to throw that punch, to hit that head – or kick that head if you're in taekwondo. It's the vision that comes first, and that comes from the brain. That's the starting point.

'If you start with vision as the most important thing, first off, and then you start to look at all other aspects, then you really begin to understand your athletes and you will actually watch them in a different manner.

'I spent so many hours watching our first team, reserve team, youth team, schoolboys, plus my own boys as well. You start to pick up the importance of the visual and cognitive aspects of the brain that are underutilised for sporting performance.'

We've seen what these aspects are. Information from the eyes feeds anticipation and high-speed decision-making. Athletes break down the blizzard of information from their senses into chunks, process it, and then decide what to do based on instinct and previous experience. It's automatic, recognition-primed decision-making.

'After a lot of thought and testing and enquiries, one day in the middle of the night I woke up and there was just this thing resounding in my ears,' remembers Clegg. 'Rapid cognition. Rapid cognition. Rapid cognition.'

Brain Training in Practice

Neuroscience is revolutionising sport by changing the way athletes train. Scientists have identified what gives athletes the edge, and are developing new training tools to hone and sharpen that advantage. The reason I've come to see Clegg is to get an idea of how these tools are used in practice; to find out whether, outside of the promotional videos and in-house research of the companies that make them, they can be integrated into an athlete's training regime to prepare them for competition.

The brain is trainable. Athletes develop their skills through thousands of hours of practice, and their brains change as they do. Neurons in the brain wire together or fall apart, and, by targeting them with clever techniques and new technologies, we can make training more efficient and maybe even break the 10,000-hour rule.

Clegg hands me a pair of 3D glasses. There's no popcorn, alas. His search for a way to train rapid cognition and decision-making in athletes eventually led him to Jocelyn Faubert, the Canadian psychologist who developed the NeuroTracker software. It's multiple-object tracking training that works much like the HELIX programme I tried at Hoffenheim, but this time with 3D depth. Eight yellow spheres appear on screen. Four of them flash orange briefly and then return to yellow, and the user's job is to track those four over a 15-second period as they move around and bounce off each other.

At the end, numbers come up and the user has to identify which four were highlighted at the start. Get them right and it speeds up for the next round. Get them wrong and it slows down. I get a score of around 1.5 – respectable, but nothing special.

Aaron Cook has recorded some of the highest scores ever seen on the NeuroTracker software, and his superiority is clear to see when he takes on Pierre, the non-league footballer who is looking to improve his game by training his brain. Cook averages around 3.5, and is able to maintain his performance even when extra challenges are added. One is called 'agility'. A motion tracker originally designed for a games console detects his position, and he has to keep his eye on the balls while jumping out of the way of a bar that comes towards him, covering half the screen. It's all about training multiple-object tracking and executive function which, as we discovered in chapter four, seems to translate into an improvement in on-field decision-making.

Clegg introduced the same brain-training software to Manchester United, where it was popular. 'We had a massive buy-in to the NeuroTracker at Man United,' he says. 'They loved it.' It has reportedly fallen out of use since the changes in management at the club, although multiple-object tracking is still mentioned during the virtual video tour you're shown if you go to Carrington.

However, the software is being more widely adopted by a number of elite sporting organisations. On the day I visit Clegg, he's also showing the equipment to a visiting sports psychologist from a top tier Australian Rules football team, which has just purchased the NeuroTracker software to use with its players.

Clegg's gym also has other tools, for training peripheral vision and speed. The Dynavision D2 does the former. It's a tall black unit with an array of small lights that pop red in a random sequence, and the athlete has to tap them when they come on – as many as they can in 60 seconds. Cook has been using this for a while and he's trained his peripheral vision to such an extent that he's able to keep his head completely still and focused on the middle of the board while his arms hit their targets, whereas Pierre, who has only been doing it for a month, has to look towards the lights to hit them accurately.

There's also the iSpan, a metal frame that reaches from floor to ceiling with lights arranged on it – three at floor level, three at chest height, and three near the top. The athletes use their hands and their feet, kicking at the lower lights and jumping up to reach the high ones. This time, the sequence stays the same each time. 'If they can learn the sequence as quickly as possible then they've got an advantage,' says Clegg.

I ask Cook, once he's finished 15 punishment press-ups for kicking one of Clegg's lights too hard, whether he thinks the training has helped his taekwondo. 'Yeah. Yeah, hugely,' he says. 'Because you can take in so much more instead of just looking at one thing; you're able to take in four or five things which gives you an advantage. All this stuff is really advanced so it's not something that you would do in normal taekwondo training.'

The challenge for coaches like Clegg, and for the designers of cognitive training tools, is to prove that the mental skills they claim to target do transfer into real-world sporting performance. Not everything works, and there are two $85,000 testaments to that standing under a tarpaulin in the middle of Clegg's gym. He pulls it back just enough to reveal a dark grey monolith, towering over us like something out of *2001: A Space Odyssey* and etched with the Nike logo and the words 'SPARQ Sensory Performance Equipment'.

'They're actually from Manchester United,' explains Clegg. 'Why are they here? Because they're never used. $85,000 that cost – designed by engineers, scientists. It didn't work. The athletes didn't want to use it; they couldn't see where it was relevant to sport. That's why, if you notice, there's a lot of stuff here that's just a ball on a string, because that's actually what you use in football – balls – so you need them as part of your training tools. It's all right spending all that money on expensive equipment but it has to be engineered with the athlete in mind.'

For Clegg, that means that training the brain is all about combining the cognitive training tools with strength or skill training; that's the only way you'll get the benefits to transfer. He calls it 'splicing', and it might involve alternating bouts of physical exercise with rounds of peripheral-vision training, or lifting weights while doing

NeuroTracker – there's a weight rack in front of the screen for that very purpose.

'You've got to make it as specific to the sport as you can,' says Clegg. One very useful and deceptively simple way of doing that is the FitLight – a wireless LED with a motion sensor attached. A set of FitLights can be arranged in any configuration, with the variety of exercises limited only by the coach's imagination. To start with, Clegg arranges eight of them in a straight line in front of the athlete, spaced out about a foot apart.

They light up in a random sequence, and the athlete has to switch them off as quickly as possible by waving a foot over them, at which point the next one lights up. It trains focus and attention, as well as footwork – ideal for both football and taekwondo.

NBA player Stephen Curry provides one example of how these brain-training tools can be spliced together with skill training. He has been pictured training using the FitLights arranged on a wall and then playing them while dribbling a basketball. He has to keep the ball under control with one hand, while using his other to trigger the light.

Clegg demonstrates another sport-specific drill. He gives Pierre a ball and arranges the lights in a large square around him. When a light turns on, the player has to dribble the ball over to that area and wave his foot over the light to switch it off as quickly as possible, and then start scanning for the next target. 'Remember, speed without control is nothing,' is Clegg's one bit of advice to the footballer before the drill starts.

Clegg believes that by tapping into what we know about the brain, and the work of scientists and software developers, he can train both speed and control. Aaron Cook has bet his Olympic dream on it.

Make Better Decisions

Some organisations are proceeding with more caution. The England and Wales Cricket Board are dipping their toe into the water of new tools for training anticipation. 'If it's specific to the brain's visual system and you can get that transferable benefit then it's worth it,' says Raph Brandon, head of science and medicine at the ECB. 'But if it's so specific that you only get better at the cognitive training tool or the computer game then you have wasted a player's time.'

There are unanswered questions. 'We're in the investigation stage,' says Brandon. 'Anticipation skills are definitely trainable, but I think it's about understanding how they are more trainable than cricket-specific training and optimising that. And at what stages of development – when you're a 12-year-old playing lots of different sports, versus when you're a 17-year-old specialising just in cricket, versus when you're a 24-year-old playing in the England team.'

The ECB and others are, however, forging ahead with other ways of training the brain.

Under pressure, athletes think too much about things that should be automatic, or get distracted by emotions and make the wrong choices in high-stakes situations. Our knowledge of the brain is helping to change this. A number of researchers whose work I've looked at are collaborating in great secrecy with sporting organisations to get athletes ready for performance under pressure. Cook will not be the only athlete at the Olympics who has trained his brain.

In cricket, they're looking at biofeedback as a way of training batsmen to deal with pressure. Instead of their brains, sensors will measure the players' heart rates, but the principle is the same. By teaching players to train and be aware of their emotional state, it's hoped they will become more resilient when the competition gets tough.

Professor Vincent Walsh, one of the world's leading cognitive neuroscientists, has also been training athletes to deal with pressure. I first met him at the GlaxoSmithKline Human Performance Lab where he was testing how elite athletes responded to physical pressure, and I spoke to him again a few months later, a couple of days after England's defeat against Wales in the 2015 Rugby World Cup. It was a result that left the hosts on the brink of elimination from the tournament in the group stages.

Towards the end of the game, England captain Chris Robshaw had a decision to make. His team were trailing, but they had won a penalty and could either take the safe option and kick the points to guarantee a draw, or go for the risky, game-winning try. Robshaw chose to go for the big score, but the team failed to complete it, and England lost the game.

'It's the second time he's made exactly that decision,' Walsh points out. 'In one of his first two or three games as captain he made exactly that kind of decision with exactly the same kind of result. There are times when your decision-making style might be great until the 77th minute, but in the 77th minute you have to be able to change your decision-making style.'

Walsh is helping athletes make better decisions under pressure.

'You're working on players' skills and players' physical abilities from a very young age and then what happens is, when people get to a very high level of performance, we start to think, "Well, maybe we should do something about their psychology." There are some Premier League teams that travel to away games with four or five physios or more. That's how seriously we take the body. But the same teams might have a psychologist working for them two days a week.' That discrepancy between body and mind in sport has been highlighted by historic attitudes towards concussions and head injuries – another area, as we've seen, that has been illuminated by recent scientific breakthroughs.

'The real differences in athletes and performances these days is in the psychology, is in the head game,' says Walsh. 'Nobody said that England, or anybody else that has lost a rugby match this past few weeks, has lost a rugby match because the players weren't muscular enough, or weren't fast enough, or weren't skilled enough. If you listen to all the commentaries, it's all about decision-making and decision-making under pressure.

'I find it hard to believe that people in multimillion-pound industries are not taking the mental side of the game seriously.'

They are starting to, though. Walsh remains sceptical of the claims of cognitive training tools, and is particularly opposed to neurofeedback and artificial brain interventions for sport. Instead, he uses technology as a diagnostic tool, to help build up a picture of what kind of decision-makers people are, so that training can be specifically targeted towards making them better.

'First of all, we profile each individual athlete,' he tells me. A profile would consist of watching the athlete in action, speaking to them and also having them complete some of the computer-based tests of decision-making under pressure. These are similar to the ones employed at the Human Performance Lab; they could involve searching for particular objects on a screen as quickly as possible, or risk-and-reward-based tasks under different kinds of pressure.

'Then we ask the athlete whether he sees anything in that profile that resonates with his game,' continues Walsh. 'We work individually with them all and ask: "Can we make this person's decision-making better at one critical point of the game, or the race, or the fight, and exactly what pressures are we trying to get this person to survive under?"

'So, if it's physical pressure, then we can set up a training routine where maybe somebody's done some intervals before they do the routine so that they're well exhausted – more exhausted than they would usually be in a race. Then we can put them through the decision-making process. We can put them in those training regimes and say, "What will you do now?"

'So when they come into that position in a competition, and they're really under pressure, it's not the first time that they're making that decision under pressure. If I would throw one criticism at what I've seen in the Rugby World Cup, and what you see at lots of international competitions, is that you see players in a situation for the first time.'

Walsh would like to see psychology and neuroscience integrated earlier into athletes' development, to make them more resilient. 'A footballer at the age of 19 or 20 will be expected to perform at his absolute best, top of his game, 40 times a year or more,' he says. 'I don't think I've had to perform at the limits of my capacities 40 times in my life. That would be one outstanding performance every year of your working life. My guess is that most of us get away without that.

'We're asking 18-, 19-, 20-year-old boys to do this under the glare of Twitter and Facebook – and that stuff matters when you're 18, 19, 20, the glare of newspapers and TV, your sponsors and your teammates and your coaches.

'Think of the pressures and the judgement these people get,' finishes Walsh. 'Even politicians only get judged once every five years. The pressures are immense, and it's actually an abdication of responsibility for people not to take on board the wealth of expertise we've got in psychology and neuroscience.

'If you can practise physical skills, and if you can practise routines and drills, you can practise the mental skills that go with them.'

The Next Sporting Revolution

The aggregation of marginal gains is a fashionable concept in sport, having been popularised by Great Britain's all-conquering cycling team under Dave Brailsford. The idea is that by paying attention to the tiniest details – instructing riders not to shake hands with anyone in the lead-up to a race so that they don't get ill, or spraying alcohol on the tyres to give them a tiny bit of extra grip before a standing start – you get the cumulative effect of lots of little improvements adding up. Athletes and teams are always looking for an edge, a small change they can make to eke out an extra 1 or 2 per cent, which in sport can be the difference between success and failure.

Our new knowledge of the brain is helping us push the limits of human performance. Unpicking the underlying factors that influence sporting ability – an innate sporting brain – could help identify people with the potential for world-class talent before they've ever kicked a ball or picked up a bat. Understanding why some people are more inclined to put their lives on the line, or how minds and bodies interact during physical exertion, can help both elite and amateur athletes push back the barriers of what's possible, while flow states could smash them entirely.

Try it in your own training, whatever your sport. Find out what experts do differently, where they look to get the advance information they need, and make your development more efficient by homing in on that area. Use the quiet eye to improve your performance in golf. Use computer programs and iPad apps to train your visual acuity or improve your ability to track multiple objects. Push the limits of your endurance by reducing your perception of effort, and improve your performance under pressure by changing the way you practise.

Neuroscience offers more than just marginal gains. The new sporting revolution has the potential to be a much more significant gain, a giant leap rather than an incremental improvement. There are moments in sporting history when progress makes huge strides forward – a better understanding of diet in football, for example, or the increased appreciation of aerodynamics in track cycling. At the top level, athletes have better nutrition and better equipment than ever before, but we're still far from maxing out the potential of the brain.

It took me a while to track down Wayne Rooney. I finally managed it in November 2015, on a morning when his head was making yet more headlines. He had scored with it in front of a packed Old Trafford the previous evening, a 79th-minute winner in a 1-0 Champions League group stage victory over CSKA Moscow. The next day, he's back at United's ground, relaxing in training kit on a leather sofa in the directors' lounge. 'I dream of the game,' he tells me, in his distinctive accent, when I ask him how he gets himself mentally ready. 'I always visualise and prepare myself the same way for every game.'

The goal involved a well-timed run into the box to meet a first-time cross from winger Jesse Lingard. Rooney had to anticipate when Lingard would get the ball into the centre, and choose the right angle of run, with the right timing. 'I think that's just about how you see the game,' he says. 'I think that's just trying to read the game and knowing the teammates as well, knowing their qualities. I obviously knew Jesse Lingard could cross the ball the way he did, so you try and put yourself in a position where you feel the ball is going to come.'

Rooney thinks he is a better decision-maker now than when he started his career as a 16-year-old at Everton. 'Naturally you learn from playing the game from when I was a young boy,' he says. 'You learn what positions to be in the older you get. When I was younger, I was a bit too eager, getting in there too quick. Now you try and be a bit more patient.'

His abilities of anticipation and decision-making have come from experience, from thousands of hours of practice. Neuroscientists and psychologists have homed in on that crucial component of sporting excellence, and are developing new training tools and technologies to target it more efficiently. They're investigating ways of speeding up neural plasticity and breaking the 10,000-hour rule, and finding out how to make athletes more resilient to choking under pressure. Our new knowledge of the brain has revealed the dangers of concussions, and could discover the next great sporting talent. It can help athletes of all ability levels push the limits of their performance, and at the elite level it's smashing down barriers and making the impossible possible.

This is the next sporting revolution.

'You need to prepare yourself for the game,' says Rooney.

'Physically *and* mentally.'

ACKNOWLEDGEMENTS

Not for the first time during this process, I don't really know where to start.

Writing a book was something I'd thought about doing eventually, but it would have remained that way for quite a while longer if not for my brilliant agent Richard Pike at Curtis Brown. He was instrumental in starting me along this path, helping me sharpen my half-formed ideas into something people might actually want to read, and getting the proposal in front of the right people. That includes my editor Ian Marshall, who saw the potential – he deserves thanks for giving a first-time writer a chance, as does everyone at Simon & Schuster for turning it from a Word document full of misused semi-colons into what you're holding now.

Of course, I wouldn't have got this far without the dozens of people who took time out of their busy schedules to speak to me. I knew I wanted to get interviews from a mixture of elite athletes and leading academics – I hadn't anticipated the latter being the more difficult to pin down.

So I'm grateful to Dr Phil Culverhouse, Dr Vincent Walsh, Professor Bruce Abernethy, Dr Nils Kolling, Jason Sada, Dr Peter Fadde, Jason Sherwin, Dr Joan Vickers, Dr Steve Bull, Dr Mark Bawden, Debbie Crews, Steven Kotler, Chris Nowinski, Ed Lodge, Raph Brandon, Professor Samuele Marcora, Robbie Britton, Billy Morgan and Simon Wheatcroft.

Special thanks are due to Dr Jan Mayer at Hoffenheim, Dr Willie Stewart, Dr Barry O'Neill at the GSK Human Performance Lab, Christina Lavelle at Brainworks, and Mick Clegg and Aaron Cook for inviting me to see things in person.

Countless people have helped set up interviews with athletes and other opportunities, but particular thanks to Adam Phillips at Wasserman and Beth Wild at the ECB.

I also need to thank my colleagues past and present at *Sport* magazine – Tony Hodson for the freedom to disappear in the middle of the day to do interviews or get my brain poked at, Sarah Shephard for leading the way and her wealth of contacts, Alex Reid for advice on first lines, Mark Coughlan for rugby quotes, and everyone else for putting up with the various tics I developed during two weeks of 'book lockdown'. Sorry for all the clicking.

This would be a much poorer book if not for the many people who I bounced ideas off, and who pored over drafts making suggestions and pointing out things that didn't make sense. Thanks to all my early readers, but particularly Edd Pickering, whose comments combined thoughtful feedback, insightful examples and jokes at my expense.

Thanks also to all my friends and family for their interest and support – especially my mum, Alka, her partner Simon, my sister Lina, and my dad Jaldeep.

Most of all, I am eternally grateful to my partner Sara for so many things – proofreading and advice, moral support and encouragement, for keeping me on track, and for putting up with me covering the dining table and the walls with notes and being even more useless than usual for a year of evenings and weekends. I couldn't have done this without you. And I promise I'll get a desk.

BIBLIOGRAPHY

In addition to the fuller list of references below, the following books and website proved particularly useful more generally, provided background information, or helped guide my thinking on certain topics.

Dan Peterson's excellent blog at axonpotential.com/blog

Bounce by Matthew Syed (London: Fourth Estate, 2011)

Choke by Sian Beilock (London: Constable & Robinson, 2011)

Faster, Higher, Stronger by Mark McClusky (New York: Plume, 2015)

Flow in Sports by Susan Jackson and Mihaliy Csikszentmihalyi (Champaign, IL: Human Kinetics, 1999)

Head Games by Christopher Nowinski (East Bridgewater, MA: Drummond Publishing, 2006)

Outliers by Malcolm Gladwell (London: Penguin Books, 2009)

Perception, Cognition, and Decision Training by Joan Vickers (Leeds: Human Kinetics Europe Ltd, 2007)

The Brain that Changes Itself by Norman Doidge (London: Penguin Books, 2008)

The Chimp Paradox by Steve Peters (London: Vermilion, 2012)

The Rise of Superman by Steven Kotler (London: Quercus, 2015)

The Sports Gene by David Epstein (London: Yellow Jersey Press, 2014)

The Talent Code by Daniel Coyle (London: Arrow Books, 2010)

Thinking Fast and Slow by Daniel Kahneman (London: Penguin Books, 2012)

NOTES AND REFERENCES

A handful of the quotes in this book are from interviews I originally conducted for *Sport* magazine. More recent pieces can be viewed at sport-magazine.co.uk

INTRODUCTION

p.1 'When a cross comes into the box, there are so many things that go through your mind in a split second' – Wayne Rooney
Winner, D. (16 May 2012). ESPN FC: Beautiful game. Beautiful mind. Retrieved 28 November 2015, from http://sports.espn.go.com/IndexPages/news/story?id=7938409

p. 2 'There was one goal that stood out' – Paul McGuinness
Bartram, S. (23 October 2008). A star is born. Retrieved 28 November 2015, from http://www.manutd.com/en/News-And-Features/Features/2008/Oct/A-star-is-born.aspx

CHAPTER ONE

p. 7 'The English team's star striker races down the left'
You can see this, and other videos of Mustachio and his robot teammates in action, on the University of Plymouth's Robot Football Facebook page: https://www.facebook.com/University-of-Plymouth-Robot-Football-148285347160/timeline/

p. 8 'you would need to use every computer in the world'
Hilbert, M. & Lopez, P. (2011). The World's Technological Capacity to Store, Communicate, and Compute Information. *Science*, 332(6025), 60-55. doi:10.1126/science.1200970

p. 11 'A series of "occlusion" studies'
Müller, S., Abernethy, B. & Farrow, D. (2006). How do world-class cricket batsmen anticipate a bowler's intention?. *The Quarterly Journal of Experimental Psychology* 59 (12), 2162-2186.

p. 11 'Abernethy has also asked squash players'
Abernethy, B. (1990). Anticipation in squash: Differences in advance cue utilization between expert and novice players. *Journal of Sports Sciences* 8 (1), 17-34.

p. 12 'Cristiano Ronaldo can score goals with his eyes shut'
The tests on Cristiano Ronaldo were conducted for a promotional documentary called *Tested to the Limits*, which is available on YouTube: https://www.youtube.com/watch?v=vSL-gPMPVXI

p. 13 'Some have a mental top speed of 80' – Xavi
Caceres, J. (July 26 2011). Dann schnapp' ich mid den Messi. *Suddeutsche Zeitung.* Translated from German.

p. 13 'This is a trait shared by the world's best passers'
Jordet, G., Heijmerikz, J. & Bloomfield, J. (March 2013). The hidden foundation of field vision in English Premier (EPL) soccer players. Paper presented at the MIT Sloan Sports Analytics Conference.

p. 13 'That's what I do: look for spaces' – Xavi
Lowe, S. (11 February 2011). I'm a romantic, says Xavi, heartbeat of Barcelona and Spain. *Guardian.* Retrieved 28 November 2015, from http://www.theguardian.com/football/2011/feb/11/xavi-barcelona-spain-interview

p. 14 'used head-mounted cameras to measure the eye movements'
Land, M. F. & Mcleod, P. (2000). From eye movements to actions: how batsmen hit the ball. *Nature Neuroscience* 3(12), 1340-1345. http://dx.doi.org/10.1038/81887

p. 16 'They were first discovered by chance in the early 1990s'
Rizzolatti, G. & Craighero, L. (2004). The mirror-neuron system. *Annual Review of Neuroscience* 27 (1), 169-192. doi:10.1146/annurev.neuro.27.070203.144230

p. 17 'The neuron is adopting the other person's point of view'
Ramachandran, V. (November 2010). The neurons that shaped civilization [Video file]. Retrieved from: https://www.ted.com/talks/vs_ramachandran_the_neurons_that_shaped_civilization?language=en
Ramachandran actually goes even further: he argues that the evolution of a mirror neuron system led directly to the sudden explosion of new skills across the human race around 75,000 to 100,000 years ago. In

short, he believes that the mirror neuron system is directly responsible for human culture as we know it.

p. 17 'A study conducted with basketball players in Rome'
Aglioti, S., Cesari, P., Romani, M., & Urgesi, C. (2008). Action anticipation and motor resonance in elite basketball players. *Nature Neuroscience* 11(9), 1109-1116. http://dx.doi.org/10.1038/nn.2182

p. 18 'tested 387 professional baseball players'
Laby, D., Davidson, J., Rosenbaum, L., Strasser, C., Mellman, M., Rosenbaum, A. & Kirschen, D. (1996). The Visual Function of Professional Baseball Players. *American Journal of Ophthalmology* 122(4), 476-485. http://dx.doi.org/10.1016/s0002-9394(14)72106-3

p. 18 'Another study compared 157 Olympic athletes'
Laby, D., Kirschen, D. & Pantall, P. (2011). The Visual Function of Olympic-Level Athletes – An Initial Report. *Eye & Contact Lens: Science & Clinical Practice* 37(3), 116-122. http://dx.doi.org/10.1097/icl.0b013e31820c5002

p. 19 'the "hardware and software" paradigm'
Epstein, D. *The Sports Gene.*
Another study found that women with good depth perception improved much more quickly when practising catching than women with poor depth perception. Because of their better depth perception 'hardware', they were able to develop their mental software much more rapidly.

p. 22 'The dorsal and ventral streams work together in sport'
Van der Kamp, J., Rivas, F., Van Doorn, H. & Savelsbergh, G. J. P. (2008). Ventral and dorsal contributions in visual anticipation in fast ball sports. *International Journal of Sport Psychology* 39(2), 100-130.

p. 22 'One study asked expert golfers to putt with their weaker side'
Johnston, A., Benton, C. P. & Nishida, S. (2003). Golfers may have to overcome a persistent visuospatial illusion. *Perception* 32, 1151-1154. doi: 10.1068/p5056

p. 24 'Researchers at University College London'
Hagura, N., Kanai, R., Orgs, G. & Haggard, P. (2012). Ready steady slow: action preparation slows the subjective passage of time. *Proceedings of the Royal Society B: Biological Sciences* 279(1746), 4399-4406. http://dx.doi.org/10.1098/rspb.2012.1339

p. 25 'Place and grid cells'
Blakeslee, S. & Blakeslee, M. (2008). *The Body Has a Mind of Its Own.* New York: Random House.

CHAPTER TWO

p. 31 'most people will be able to remember around seven items and then struggle'
One of the interesting ways of measuring how taxing a mental task is on working memory is by looking at the dilation of the pupil – the harder the task, the more dilated it gets. This is called cognitive pupilometry, and it's discussed at length in Daniel Kahneman's *Thinking Fast and Slow.*

p. 33 'Adriaan de Groot ran an innovative experiment'
Brook, C. & de Groot, A. (1966). Thought and Choice in Chess. *The American Journal of Psychology* 79(2), 348. http://dx.doi.org/10.2307/1421155

p. 33 'Another study of chess players'
Chase, W. & Simon, H. (1973). Perception in chess. *Cognitive Psychology* 4(1), 55-81. http://dx.doi.org/10.1016/0010-0285(73)90004-2

p. 33 'knocked off their perch'
Williams, M., Davids, K., Burwitz, L. & Williams, J. (1993). Cognitive knowledge and soccer performance. *Perceptual and Motor Skills* 76(2), 579-593. http://dx.doi.org/10.2466/pms.1993.76.2.579

p. 34 'High school American football coaches'
Garland, D. & Barry, J. (1991). Cognitive Advantage in Sport: The Nature of Perceptual Structures. *The American Journal of Psychology* 104(2), 211. http://dx.doi.org/10.2307/1423155

p. 34 'A lot of coaches use numbering systems' – Trent Dilfer
Method Men: How NFL Players Memorize Dizzying Playbooks. (2011). Retrieved 29 November 2015, from http://forum.go-bengals.com/index.php?/topic/58998-method-men-how-nfl-players-memorize-dizzying-playbooks/

p. 35 'asked a group of footballers to dribble through a slalom course'
Smith, M. & Chamberlin, C. (1992). Effect of adding cognitively demanding tasks on soccer skill performance. *Perceptual and Motor Skills* 75(3), 955-961. http://dx.doi.org/10.2466/pms.1992.75.3.955

p. 35 'Further down the California coast'
Wymbs, N., Bassett, D., Mucha, P., Porter, M. & Grafton, S. (2012). Differential Recruitment of the Sensorimotor Putamen and Frontoparietal Cortex during Motor Chunking in Humans. *Neuron* 74(5), 936-946. http://dx.doi.org/10.1016/j.neuron.2012.03.038

p. 37 'analysed over 2.5 million golf putts'
Pope, D. & Schweitzer, M. (2011). Is Tiger Woods Loss Averse? Persistent

Bias in the Face of Experience, Competition, and High Stakes. *American Economic Review* 101(1), 129-157. http://dx.doi.org/10.1257/aer.101.1.129

p. 39 'Kolling and his colleagues at Oxford'
Kolling, N., Wittmann, M. & Rushworth, M. (2014). Multiple Neural Mechanisms of Decision Making and Their Competition under Changing Risk Pressure. *Neuron* 81(5), 1190-1202. http://dx.doi.org/10.1016/j.neuron.2014.01.033

p. 40 'a wide range of brain regions across the frontal and parietal lobes'
Yarrow, K., Brown, P. & Krakauer, J. (2009). Inside the brain of an elite athlete: the neural processes that support high achievement in sports. *Nature Reviews Neuroscience* 10(8), 585-596. http://dx.doi.org/10.1038/nrn2672

p. 40 'The brain does not merely issue rigid commands'
Zimmer, C. (2010). The Brain: Why Athletes Are Geniuses. *Discover.* Retrieved from: http://discovermagazine.com/2010/apr/16-the-brain-athletes-are-geniuses

p. 41 'a simple procedure that helps find adequate, though often imperfect, answers to difficult questions'
Kahneman also points out that the word heuristic shares the same etymological root as 'eureka', which is nice.

p. 41 'Used a bowling machine to test what approach skilled fielders in cricket use'
McLeod, P. & Dienes, Z. (1996). Do fielders know where to go to catch the ball or only how to get there? *Journal of Experimental Psychology: Human Perception and Performance* 22(3), 531-543. http://dx.doi.org/10.1037//0096-1523.22.3.531

p. 43 'covered the eyes of American footballers'
Shaffer, D., Dolgov, I., Mcmanama, E., Swank, C., Maynor, A., Kelly, K. & Neuhoff, J. (2013). Blind(fold)ed by science: A constant target-heading angle is used in visual and nonvisual pursuit. *Psychonomic Bulletin & Review* 20(5), 923-934. http://dx.doi.org/10.3758/s13423-013-0412-5

p. 44 'to make the unpredictable world of sport predictable'
'Indeed, the purpose of extensive training is to make much of the unpredictable world of sport predictable, and therefore something that can be controlled more easily,' writes Joan Vickers in *Perception, Cognition, and Decision Training.*

CHAPTER THREE

The original research which spawned the hotly debated 10,000 hours rule.
Ericsson himself says Gladwell misconstrued his research:

Ericsson, K., Krampe, R. & Tesch-Romer, C. (1993). The role of deliberate practice in the acquisition of expert performance. *Psychological Review* 100(3), 363-406. http://dx.doi.org/10.1037/0033-295x.100.3.363
Gladwell, M. *Outliers*.

p. 48 'No matter how many hours of practice you put in'
Although that's not to say that you're guaranteed to be good at sprinting, regardless of your genes. Daniel Coye's book *The Talent Code* points out that the world's best sprinters tend to have older siblings: the idea being that having someone slightly faster than them tends to spur them on.

p. 49 'The plastic brain is like a snowy hill in winter' – Alvaro Pascual-Leone
Doidge, N. *The Brain that Changes Itself.*

p. 51 'black cabbies in the English capital'
Maguire, E., Gadian, D., Johnsrude, I., Good, C., Ashburner, J., Frackowiak, R. & Frith, C. (2000). Navigation-related structural change in the hippocampi of taxi drivers. *Proceedings of the National Academy of Sciences* 97(8), 4398-4403. http://dx.doi.org/10.1073/pnas.070039597

p. 51 'Golfers come in all shapes and sizes'
Jäncke, L., Koeneke, S., Hoppe, A., Rominger, C. & Hänggi, J. (2009). The Architecture of the Golfer's Brain. *PLoS ONE* 4(3), e4785. http://dx.doi.org/10.1371/journal.pone.0004785

p. 52 'had started at a much younger age'
13.1 compared to 14.5 for the 1-14 handicapped group, and 19 for the 15-36 handicapped group.

p. 52 'compared the brains of professional divers with those of non-divers'
Wei, G., Zhang, Y., Jiang, T. & Luo, J. (2011). Increased Cortical Thickness in Sports Experts: A Comparison of Diving Players with the Controls. *PLoS ONE* 6(2), e17112. http://dx.doi.org/10.1371/journal.pone.0017112

p. 53 'They scanned the brains of jugglers' Draganski, B., Gaser, C., Busch, V., Schuierer, G., Bogdahn, U. & May, A. (2004). Neuroplasticity: Changes in grey matter induced by training. *Nature* 427(6972), 311-312. http://dx.doi.org/10.1038/427311a

p. 56 'There was no prodding the virtuosos with electrodes while they played'
Elbert, T., Pantev, C., Wienbruch, C., Rockstroh, B. & Taub, E. (1995). Increased Cortical Representation of the Fingers of the Left Hand in String Players. *Science* 270(5234), 305-307. http://dx.doi.org/10.1126/science.270.5234.305

p. 57 'Rackets are the most important thing for a tennis player,'
Bishop, G. (2014). Seeking Bigger Sweet Spot, Roger Federer Hopes His Racket Will Grow on Him. Nytimes.com. Retrieved 29 November 2015,

from http://www.nytimes.com/2014/01/17/sports/tennis/is-change-good-federer-with-new-racket-to-find-out.html?_r=0

p. 59 'Coley took time out to show me where to live, showed me all the places to go' – Dwight Yorke

Manutd.com.The Yorke & Cole show: 15 years on – Official Manchester United Website. Retrieved 29 November 2015, from http://www.manutd.com/en/News-And-Features/United-Uncovered/News/2013/Aug/Issue-27/video-interview-dwight-yorke-and-andy-cole-on-Treble-season.aspx

p. 61 'learn to use your muscles more efficiently'

A group of scientists in Colorado discovered that even when volunteers had mastered a task, in this case controlling a robotic arm, there were still energy savings to be had because of the increasing efficiency of the brain. When you learn a new motor skill, your cortical map for that area of the body grows, but eventually you need fewer neurons to do the job because you learn to use your muscles more efficiently.

Another study, by neurobiologist Professor Peter Strick at the University of Pittsburgh, trained monkeys to complete two different tasks: one they learnt and repeated from memory, and another that required them to respond to a point appearing on a screen. They showed the same level of neurons firing in both tasks, but the memorised task took up less energy because they already knew how to do it.

p. 61 'examine how much more efficient all that practice had made Neymar's brain'

Naito, E. & Hirose, S. (2014). Efficient foot motor control by Neymar's brain. *Frontiers in Human Neuroscience* 8. http://dx.doi.org/10.3389/fnhum.2014.00594

p. 63 'It's one of the most intricate and exquisite cell-to-cell processes there is' – Dr Douglas Fields

Coyle, D. *The Talent Code.*

p. 65 'causing me to think of BDNF as Miracle-Gro for the brain'

Ratey, J. & Hagerman, E. (2008). *Spark!* New York: Little, Brown.

p. 66 'You have a blank period during World War I. Then a blank period during World War II. And then one during World War Lance.' – Lance Armstrong

Okbo, M. & Sorensen, J. (2014). *Rouleur* (52).

p. 67 'One study of amateur triathletes in Germany'

Dietz, P., Ulrich, R., Dalaker, R., Striegel, H., Franke, A., Lieb, K. & Simon, P. (2013). Associations between Physical and Cognitive Doping – A Cross-Sectional Study in 2.997 Triathletes. *PLoS ONE* 8(11), e78702. http://dx.doi.org/10.1371/journal.pone.0078702

p. 68 'Neuroscientists at Johns Hopkins University'
Reis, J., Schambra, H., Cohen, L., Buch, E., Fritsch, B. & Zarahn, E. et al. (2009). Noninvasive cortical stimulation enhances motor skill acquisition over multiple days through an effect on consolidation. *Proceedings of the National Academy of Sciences* 106(5), 1590-1595. http://dx.doi.org/10.1073/pnas.0805413106

p. 68 'may also be found in the gym of athletes training for the Olympics or alternatively on the list of illegitimate doping remedies'
Nielsen, J. & Cohen, L. (2008). The olympic brain. Does corticospinal plasticity play a role in acquisition of skills required for high-performance sports? *The Journal of Physiology* 586(1), 65-70. http://dx.doi.org/10.1113/jphysiol.2007.142661

p. 69 'The researchers had reopened the window for rapid learning'
This is discussed at length in *The Brain that Changes Itself* but the key paper is: Kilgard, M. (1998). Cortical Map Reorganization Enabled by Nucleus Basalis Activity. *Science* 279(5357), 1714-1718. http://dx.doi.org/10.1126/science.279.5357.1714

p. 69 'injecting BDNF directly into the brain'
Rex, C., Lin, C., Kramar, E., Chen, L., Gall, C. & Lynch, G. (2007). Brain-Derived Neurotrophic Factor Promotes Long-Term Potentiation-Related Cytoskeletal Changes in Adult Hippocampus. *Journal of Neuroscience* 27(11), 3017-3029. http://dx.doi.org/10.1523/jneurosci.4037-06.2007

CHAPTER FOUR

p. 75 'Mustafa Amini stands, ready'
Video footage of Amini in action can be seen here: https://www.youtube.com/watch?v=V62MAqUP0TI

p. 76 Mario Gotze's reaction to the Footbonaut is in the video here: http://www.uefa.com/trainingground/coaches/video/videoid=1936054.html

p. 76 'A Footbonaut goal'
Rafael Honigstein points this out in his book, *Das Reboot.*

p. 78 'We brought out the training boards' – Bill Shankly
Hunter, S. (2013). How Bill Shankly changed training. Liverpool FC. Retrieved 29 November 2015, from http://www.liverpoolfc.com/news/first-team/144161-how-bill-shankly-changed-training

p. 79 'risk of smashed windows'
There are other, more outlandish types of training equipment for football as well. The Heads Up vest is a wedge-shaped bib that stops young players looking at their feet when they're on the ball, encouraging them to learn

how to control and dribble with their heads up so they can spot passes.

p. 79 'six times as many'
Benefits of Futsal (1st ed.). Retrieved from: http://www.ecfa.org.uk/media/20524/fa-futsal-benefits-guidance-resource.pdf

p. 83 'It was part of our routine because it was sort of forced on us'
BostonGlobe.com. (2015). Neuroscouting may give Red Sox a heads-up on prospects' potential. Retrieved 29 November 2015, from https://www.bostonglobe.com/sports/2015/02/18/neuroscouting-may-give-red-sox-heads-prospects-potential/EFBHR3zNdThk1NboRpNMHL/story.html

p. 84 'Oh, you have to do neuroscience or you're going to get fined'
Costa, B. (2015). Baseball's Science Experiment. *WSJ*. Retrieved 29 November 2015, from http://www.wsj.com/articles/baseballs-science-experiment-1411135882

p. 85 'paid £5 for their co-operation'
'That was totally not worth it,' was one participant's assessment at the end of the experiment.

p. 87 'Players don't want to wear something that looks like a Hydra on their heads'
Schonbrun, Z. (2015). Can two entrepreneurs turn neuroscience into Moneyball? SBNation.com. Retrieved 29 November 2015, from http://www.sbnation.com/longform/2015/7/15/8952915/take-me-out-to-the-brain-game

p. 91 'youth players from a top division Dutch football club'
Verburgh, L., Scherder, E., van Lange, P. & Oosterlaan, J. (2014). Executive Functioning in Highly Talented Soccer Players. *PLoS ONE* 9(3), e91254. http://dx.doi.org/10.1371/journal.pone.0091254

p. 91 'where he and colleagues tested 87 of their best players on their executive function'
Alves, H., Voss, M., Boot, W., Deslandes, A., Cossich, V., Salles, J. & Kramer, A. (2013). Perceptual-Cognitive Expertise in Elite Volleyball Players. *Frontiers in Psychology* 4. http://dx.doi.org/10.3389/fpsyg.2013.00036

p. 92 'The last test I found impossible'
Kuper, S. (1994). *Football Against the Enemy*. London: Orion.

p. 95 'Faubert and his colleagues used NeuroTracker to test and train 102 professional athletes'
Faubert, J. (2013). Professional athletes have extraordinary skills for rapidly learning complex and neutral dynamic visual scenes. *Sci. Rep.* 3. http://dx.doi.org/10.1038/srep01154

p. 95 'We separated the soccer players into groups'
Fitzpatrick, R. Messi and the machine.*The Blizzard* (17).

p. 96 'Every rider trains their muscles but few train their brain' – Mark Cavendish
Financial Times. (2015). Interview: British cycling star Mark Cavendish – FT.com. Retrieved 29 November 2015, from http://www.ft.com/cms/s/2/699b70fa-146c-11e5-ad6e-00144feabdc0.html

p. 96 'war simulation game *Medal of Honor*'
Boot, W., Kramer, A., Simons, D., Fabiani, M. & Gratton, G. (2008). The effects of video game playing on attention, memory, and executive control. *Acta Psychologica* 129(3), 387-398. http://dx.doi.org/10.1016/j.actpsy.2008.09.005

p. 97 'A survey of over 10,000 players at the FIFA Interactive World Cup'
FIFA.com. (2012). FIFA Interactive World Cup welcomes its millionth player. Retrieved 29 November 2015, from http://www.fifa.com/interactiveworldcup/news/y=2012/m=3/news=fifa-interactive-world-cup-welcomes-its-millionth-player-1602425.html

p. 97 'awareness of other players on the pitch'
In American football, the Madden series of games has been credited with improving tactical awareness among young players.

p. 99 'I'd never even power-steered a car before' – Jann Mardenborough
Richards, G. (2012). From gamer to racing driver. *Guardian*. Retrieved 29 November 2015, from http://www.theguardian.com/sport/2012/apr/29/jann-ardenborough-racing-car-games

CHAPTER FIVE

p. 103 'improving the way players use their eyes can improve both the quality'
Slater, C. (2015). Tributes for Manchester United doctor Gail Stephenson. *Manchester Evening News*. Retrieved 29 November 2015, from http://www.manchestereveningnews.co.uk/news/greater-manchester-news/gail-stephenson-manchester-united-vision-9694234

p. 104 'We're using the brain as glasses'
Collins, N. (2011). New iPhone app could delay need for reading glasses. Telegraph.co.uk. Retrieved 29 November 2015, from http://www.telegraph.co.uk/news/science/science-news/8794225/New-iPhone-app-could-delay-need-for-reading-glasses.html

p. 104 'Before the 2013 college baseball season'
Miller, B. Better Batters Result from Brain-training Research. *UCR Today*. Retrieved 29 November 2015, from http://ucrtoday.ucr.edu/20511

p. 105 'stroboscopic training does seem to enhance vision and attention'

Appelbaum, L., Cain, M., Schroeder, J., Darling, E. & Mitroff, S. (2013). Improving visual cognition through stroboscopic training. *Journal of Vision* 13(9), 603-603. http://dx.doi.org/10.1167/13.9.603

p. 106 'two groups of professional ice hockey players from the Carolina Hurricanes'

Mitroff, S., Friesen, P., Bennett, D., Yoo, H. & Reichow, A. (2013). Enhancing Ice Hockey Skills Through Stroboscopic Visual Training: A Pilot Study. *Athletic Training & Sports Health Care* 5(6), 261-264. http://dx.doi.org/10.3928/19425864-20131030-02

p. 106 'It is mainly for the receivers training to focus'

Borel, B. (2014). What will sports look like in the future? ideas.ted.com. Retrieved 29 November 2015, from http://ideas.ted.com/what-will-sports-look-like-in-the-future-three-ted-experts-discuss/

Chris Kluwe

http://ideas.ted.com/what-will-sports-look-like-in-the-future-three-ted-experts-discuss/

p. 107 In-depth discussion of the quiet eye:

Vickers, J. *Perception, Cognition, and Decision Training.*

p. 110 'Mike Cammalleri looks like a man possessed'

Remarkable video of Mike Cammalleri's visualisation routine can be seen here: https://www.youtube.com/watch?v=_AH2NhZhJRo

p. 111 'Part of my preparation is I go and ask the kit man what colour we're wearing' – Wayne Rooney

Winner, D. (16 May 2012). ESPN FC: Beautiful game. Beautiful mind. Retrieved 28 November 2015, from http://sports.espn.go.com/IndexPages/news/story?id=7938409

p. 111 'I use visualisation to think about the perfect technique' – Jessica Ennis-Hill

Stylist magazine. Jessica Ennis wins gold. Retrieved 29 November 2015, from http://www.stylist.co.uk/people/interviews-and-profiles/interview-jessica-ennis

p. 111 'I visualise the ball travelling along that path'

Jackson, J. (2003). How to be the best kicker in the world. *Guardian.* Retrieved 29 November 2015, from http://www.theguardian.com/sport/2003/oct/05/rugbyworldcup2003.rugbyunion13

p. 111 'a study conducted by Soviet sports psychologists'

Garfield, C. & Bennett, H. (1985). *Peak Performance.* New York, NY: Warner Books.

p. 112 'has now taken his visualisation techniques to the business world'

Bull, S. (2006). *The Game Plan.* Chichester: Capstone.

p. 113 'simply thinking about playing a sequence of keys had long-term changes to their cortical maps'
Pascual-Leone, A. (September 1995). Modulation of muscle responses evoked by transcranial magnetic stimulation during the acquisition of new fine motor skills. *Journal of Neurophysiology* 74(3), 1037-1045.

p. 113 'simply thinking about lifting weights'
Ranganathan, V., Siemionow, V., Liu, J., Sahgal, V. & Yue, G. (2004). From mental power to muscle power – gaining strength by using the mind. *Neuropsychologia* 42(7), 944-956. http://dx.doi.org/10.1016/j.neuropsychologia.2003.11.018

p. 113 'A study of elite high jumpers'
Guillot, A., Moschberger, K. & Collet, C. (2013). Coupling movement with imagery as a new perspective for motor imagery practice. *Behavioral and Brain Functions* 9(1), 8. http://dx.doi.org/10.1186/1744-9081-9-8

p. 114 'multiple-object tracking on computer training software'
Romeas, T., Guldner, A. & Faubert, J. (2016). 3D-Multiple Object Tracking training task improves passing decision-making accuracy in soccer players. *Psychology of Sport and Exercise* 22, 1-9. http://dx.doi.org/10.1016/j.psychsport.2015.06.002

p. 115 'He has given me that crucial extra metre in my head that is so important' – Dries Mertens
Sinnott, J. (2011). Cracking coaching's final frontier. News.bbc.co.uk. Retrieved 29 November 2015, from http://news.bbc.co.uk/sport1/hi/football/9421702.stm

p. 116 'When he was a boy in Belgium, he changed regularly from one club to another'
Ellis, R. (2011). Liverpool star turns to mind guru to help him adjust after big-money move. *Daily Mirror.* Retrieved 29 November 2015, from http://www.mirror.co.uk/sport/football/news/liverpools-christian-benteke-asks-mind-6387638?

p. 116 'Overload exercises help the player speed up the feet and the thought process'
Sinnott, J. The head case. *The Blizzard* (3).

p. 116 'those employed by baseball coach Joe Maddon'
Keri, J. (2011). *The Extra 2%*. New York: Ballantine Books.

p. 117 'We try to catch different shape balls' – Petr Cech
http://www.standard.co.uk/sport/football/petr-cech-reveals-the-secrets-behind-his-record-breaking-success-at-arsenal-and-chelsea-a3149711.html

CHAPTER SIX

p. 121 'The first punch was instinct'
McRae, D. (2015). Ben Flower: Every single day I regret my brutal attack on Lance Hohaia. *Guardian*. Retrieved 29 November 2015, from http://www.theguardian.com/sport/2015/apr/13/ben-flower-lance-hohaia-wigan-st-helens-grand-final-super-league-sent-off-punch-ban-regret

p. 121 'The adrenaline levels in a game can be so high' – Luis Suarez
Suarez, L., Jenson, P. & Lowe, S. (2014). *Crossing the Line*. London: Headline.

p. 122 'of Zinedine Zidane's infamous head butt in the 2006 World Cup final, of Eric Cantona's assault on a fan at Selhurst Park in 1996'
Both Cantona and Zidane have said they don't regret their actions, but we can probably interpret this as post-rationalisation/Gallic flair.

p. 124 'England's penalty shoot-out record'
Jordet, G. (2009). Why do English players fail in soccer penalty shootouts? A study of team status, self-regulation, and choking under pressure. *Journal of Sports Sciences* 27(2), 97-106. http://dx.doi.org/10.1080/02640410802509144

p. 124 'male volunteers to walk across rope bridges'
Dutton, D. & Aron, A. (1974). Some evidence for heightened sexual attraction under conditions of high anxiety. *Journal of Personality and Social Psychology* 30(4), 510-517. http://dx.doi.org/10.1037/h0037031

p. 124 'The Human and the Chimp'
Peters, S. *The Chimp Paradox*.

p. 125 'A small step to the right ruined Moacyr Barbosa's life'
This is one of 19 stories in a series of articles I wrote for *Sport* in the run-up to the 2014 World Cup. They're collected as an ebook called *World Cup Stories*.

p. 127 'It was probably the lowest point of every single one of the Brazilian players involved' – Fernandinho
Duarte, F. (2014). Fernandinho: We will have to answer questions about that game for the rest of our lives. *Guardian*. Retrieved 29 November 2015, from http://www.theguardian.com/world/2014/dec/14/fernandinho-faces-2014-brazil-answer-questions-game-rest-lives

p. 127 'Choking is suboptimal performance'
Beilock, S. *Choke*.

p. 128 'trawled through the archives of championship games'
Baumeister, R. & Steinhilber, A. (1984). Paradoxical effects of supportive audiences on performance under pressure: The

home field disadvantage in sports championships. *Journal of Personality and Social Psychology* 47(1), 85-93. http://dx.doi.org/10.1037/0022-3514.47.1.85

p. 129 'asked people to play a computer game called *Sky Jinks*'

Butler, J. & Baumeister, R. (1998). The trouble with friendly faces: Skilled performance with a supportive audience. *Journal of Personality and Social Psychology* 75(5), 1213-1230. http://dx.doi.org/10.1037//0022-3514.75.5.1213

p. 129 'People are also more likely to choke when there's something at stake'

Baumeister, R. (1984). Choking under pressure: Self-consciousness and paradoxical effects of incentives on skillful performance. *Journal of Personality and Social Psychology* 46(3), 610-620. http://dx.doi.org/10.1037//0022-3514.46.3.610

p. 130 'participants had their brain activity scanned'

Mobbs, D., Hassabis, D., Seymour, B., Marchant, J., Weiskopf, N., Dolan, R. & Frith, C. (2009). Choking on the Money: Reward-Based Performance Decrements Are Associated With Midbrain Activity. *Psychological Science* 20(8), 955-962. http://dx.doi.org/10.1111/j.1467-9280.2009.02399.x

p. 130 'Another fMRI study at Caltech'

Chib, V., De Martino, B., Shimojo, S. & O'Doherty, J. (2012). Neural Mechanisms Underlying Paradoxical Performance for Monetary Incentives Are Driven by Loss Aversion. *Neuron* 74(3), 582-594. http://dx.doi.org/10.1016/j.neuron.2012.02.038

Lehrer, J. (2012). The New Neuroscience of Choking. *New Yorker*. Retrieved 29 November 2015, from http://www.newyorker.com/tech/frontal-cortex/the-new-neuroscience-of-choking

p. 131 'Would it have all been different if Neymar had been fit?'

Jordet, G. (2009). When Superstars Flop: Public Status and Choking Under Pressure in International Soccer Penalty Shootouts. *Journal of Applied Sport Psychology* 21(2), 125-130. http://dx.doi.org/10.1080/10413200902777263

p. 132 'When I saw Luka Modric walking to the penalty spot, I knew he was going to miss'

Arbouw, E. (2008). When Superstars Flop. *UK-sportivo* (38), 24. Retrieved from: http://issuu.com/rftlapoutre/docs/uk38/24

p. 134 'asked people to tackle a climbing wall'

Pijpers, J., Oudejans, R., Holsheimer, F. & Bakker, F. (2003). Anxiety–performance relationships in climbing: a process-oriented approach. *Psychology of Sport and Exercise* 4(3), 283-304. http://dx.doi.org/10.1016/s1469-0292(02)00010-9

p. 134 'I didn't make the saves I should have made' – Sian Beilock
The University of Chicago. (2010). Brain key to 'choking' under pressure. Retrieved 29 November 2015, from http://www.uchicago.edu/features/20101025_choke/

p. 134 'she asked expert and novice footballers'
Beilock, S., Carr, T., MacMahon, C. & Starkes, J. (2002). When paying attention becomes counterproductive: Impact of divided versus skill-focused attention on novice and experienced performance of sensorimotor skills. *Journal of Experimental Psychology: Applied* 8(1), 6-16. http://dx.doi.org/10.1037//1076-898x.8.1.6

p. 135 'found a similar phenomenon with college baseball players'
Gray, R. (2004). Attending to the Execution of a Complex Sensorimotor Skill: Expertise Differences, Choking, and Slumps. *Journal of Experimental Psychology: Applied* 10(1), 42-54. http://dx.doi.org/10.1037/1076-898x.10.1.42

p. 135 'It seizes control again (with the left hemisphere particularly culpable)'
Jueptner, M., Stephan, K. M., Frith, C. D., Brooks, D. J., Frackowiak, R. S. & Passingham, R. E. (1997). Anatomy of motor learning. I. Frontal cortex and attention to action. *Journal of Neurophysiology* 77(3), 1313-1324.

p. 136 'Standing on the tee of the final hole on Sunday'
SI.com. (1999). The curious case of Jean Van de Velde's British Open disaster. *Sports Illustrated.* Retrieved 29 November 2015, from http://www.si.com/more-sports/2011/09/14/jean-vandevelde

p. 137 'Sports aren't cognitively static'
Dobbs, D. (2010). The Tight Collar: The New Science of Choking Under Pressure. *WIRED.* Retrieved 29 November 2015, from http://www.wired.com/2010/09/the-tight-collar-the-new-science-of-choking/

p. 140 'It was going to be one of the best days of my life'
Bull, A. (2013). 'It took 10 years to recover': the story of Scott Boswell and the yips. *Guardian*. Retrieved 29 November 2015, from http://www.theguardian.com/sport/2013/sep/18/scott-boswell-and-the-yips

p. 141 'She has used a device called the CyberGlove'
Owen, D. (2014). The Yips. *New Yorker.* Retrieved 29 November 2015, from http://www.newyorker.com/magazine/2014/05/26/the-yips

p. 142 'On some shots I don't even get the cue through'
News.bbc.co.uk. (2010). Hendry reveals 10-year battle with the 'yips'. Retrieved 29 November 2015, from http://news.bbc.co.uk/sport1/hi/other_sports/snooker/9267691.stm

CHAPTER SEVEN

p. 146 'I really don't think we are born being able to thrive or succeed versus fail under pressure'

The Choke. (2015). Radio 4. Retrieved from http://www.bbc.co.uk/programmes/b05v6d35

p. 147 'filming golfers during their practice sessions'

Beilock, S. & Carr, T. (2001). On the fragility of skilled performance: What governs choking under pressure? *Journal of Experimental Psychology: General* 130(4), 701-725. http://dx.doi.org/10.1037/0096-3445.130.4.701

p. 147 'asking athletes to squeeze a ball in their left hand'

Beckmann, J., Gröpel, P. & Ehrlenspiel, F. (2013). Preventing motor skill failure through hemisphere-specific priming: Cases from choking under pressure. *Journal of Experimental Psychology: General* 142(3), 679-691. http://dx.doi.org/10.1037/a0029852

p. 149 'asking people to focus their attention externally rather than internally'

Wulf, G., Höss, M. & Prinz, W. (1998). Instructions for Motor Learning: Differential Effects of Internal Versus External Focus of Attention. *Journal of Motor Behavior* 30(2), 169-179. http://dx.doi.org/10.1080/00222899809601334

p. 152 'Decision-training model'

There's a lot more on decision training in Joan Vickers' book *Perception, Cognition, and Decision Training.* She's working on an updated version.

p. 153 'high-leverage practice'

You can see the videos in question on Daniel Coyle's website: http://thetalentcode.com/2014/11/24/the-power-of-high-leverage-practice/

p. 154 'adults were better at learning a new language'

Cochran, B., McDonald, J. & Parault, S. (1999). Too Smart for Their Own Good: The Disadvantage of a Superior Processing Capacity for Adult Language Learners. *Journal of Memory and Language* 41(1), 30-58. http://dx.doi.org/10.1006/jmla.1999.2633

p. 154 'Bruce Abernethy has conducted experiments with tennis players'

Farrow, D. & Abernethy, B. (2002). Can anticipatory skills be learned through implicit video based perceptual training? *Journal of Sports Sciences* 20(6), 471-485. http://dx.doi.org/10.1080/02640410252925143

p. 156 'Marco Materazzi's comment to French talisman Zinedine Zidane'

The story behind this incident: The Italian had been persistently tugging Zidane's shirt throughout the game, and when Zidane offered to give him the shirt after the final whistle, Materazzi apparently replied: 'I would prefer your sister.'

p. 157 'A study of crucial field goal kicks in the 2002 and 2003 NFL seasons'
Berry, S. M. & Wood, C. (2004). A Statistician Reads the Sports Pages: The Cold-Foot Effect. *Chance* 17(4), 47-51.

CHAPTER EIGHT

p. 163 'I felt I could run all day without tiring' – Pele
Murphy, M. & White, R. (1995). *In the Zone*. New York: Penguin/Arkana.

p. 163 'I witnessed visibly and audibly'
Hamilton, M. *McLaren*. London: Blink

p. 164 'I realised how few of the grown-ups that I knew'
Csikszentmihalyi, M. (2004). Flow, the secret to happiness. Lecture, TED2005. Retrieved from: https://www.ted.com/talks/mihaly_csikszentmihalyi_on_flow?language=en

p. 164 'The best moments usually occur when'
Csikszentmihalyi, M. (2002). *Flow*. London: Rider.

p. 165 'Flow has been reported by runners'
Jackson, S. & Csikszentmihalyi, M. *Flow in Sports*.

p. 165 'and 48 per cent of other people'
This stat comes from research and online surveys conducted by Steven Kotler's Flow Genome Project. Find out more at flowgenomeproject.co

p. 165 'The person I became on Neva'
Schultheis, R. (1984). *Bone Games*. New York: Random House.

p. 167 'There are thought to be 17 triggers for flow in all'
They are: focused attention, clear goals, immediate feedback, the challenge/skills ratio, high consequences, rich environment, deep embodiment, serious concentration, shared goals, good communication, familiarity, equal participation and skill level, risk, a sense of control, close listening, always saying yes, and creativity.

p. 169 'Jake Marshall has been wired up like the Terminator'
This section is based on research conducted by Red Bull. You can read a summary here: http://spectrum.ieee.org/tech-talk/biomedical/imaging/neuroscience-gets-radical-how-to-study-surfers-brain-waves

p. 170 'One study of novice and expert shooters'
Deeny, S., Hillman, C., Janelle, C. & Hatfield, B. (2001). EEG coherence and neural efficiency in expert and non-expert marksmen. *Medicine & Science in Sports & Exercise* 33(5), S177. http://dx.doi.org/10.1097/00005768-200105001-01008

p. 170 'Another study of karate and fencing'
Babiloni, C., Marzano, N., Infarinato, F., Iacoboni, M., Rizza, G. &

Aschieri, P. et al. (2010). Neural efficiency of experts' brain during judgment of actions: A high-resolution EEG study in elite and amateur karate athletes. *Behavioural Brain Research* 207(2), 466-475. http://dx.doi.org/10.1016/j.bbr.2009.10.034

p. 170 'One study of darts players'
Chen, J. et al. (August 2005). Effects of anxiety on EEG coherence during dart throw. Paper presented at the meeting of the 2005 World Congress, International Society for Sport Psychology, Sydney, Australia.

p. 170 'Think of a factory'
Kotler, S. *The Rise of Superman.*

p. 171 'Seven Tibetan Buddhists and some nuns'
Newberg, A., Alavi, A., Baime, M., Pourdehnad, M., Santanna, J. & d'Aquili, E. (2001). The measurement of regional cerebral blood flow during the complex cognitive task of meditation: a preliminary SPECT study. *Psychiatry Research: Neuroimaging* 106(2), 113-122.

p. 173 'An fMRI study of jazz musicians and freestyle rappers'
Liu, S., Chow, H., Xu, Y., Erkkinen, M., Swett, K. & Eagle, M. et al. (2012). Neural Correlates of Lyrical Improvisation: An fMRI Study of Freestyle Rap. *Sci. Rep.* 2. http://dx.doi.org/10.1038/srep00834

p. 182 'I think everyone plays their best tennis when they are relaxed'
Tennishead.net. (2015). Neuroscience: Inside Mike Bryan's brain. *tennishead.* Retrieved 29 November 2015, from http://www.tennishead.net/news/academy/2015/08/17/inside-mike-bryans-brain

p. 183 'Fascinating bit of research using neurofeedback'
Berka, Chris, et al. (2010). Accelerating training using interactive neuro-educational technologies: applications to archery, golf, and rifle marksmanship. *International Journal of Sport and Society* 1 (4), 87-104.

p. 187 'In jazz, the group has the ideas'
Sawyer, R. (2007). *Group Genius.* New York: Basic Books.

p. 187 'compared solitary flow, co-active flow'
Walker, C. (2010). Experiencing flow: Is doing it together better than doing it alone? *The Journal of Positive Psychology* 5(1), 3-11. http://dx.doi.org/10.1080/17439760903271116

p. 187 'The best players are the quickest thinkers'
FourFourTwo. (2010). Andres Iniesta: How to boss the midfield. Retrieved 29 November 2015, from http://www.fourfourtwo.com/performance/training/andres-iniesta-how-boss-midfield#:VaN3bGYTgi-WNA

p. 188 'heart-rate synchrony'
Slides from McCaffrey and Bickart's presentation available here: http://www.sloansportsconference.com/?p=10448

CHAPTER NINE

p. 195 'Just keep moving forward'
You can see the Robbie Britton video here: https://www.youtube.com/watch?v=G0X0yNLRG74

p. 196 'experienced orienteers'
Hancock, S. & McNaughton, L. (1986). Effects of fatigue on ability to process visual information by experienced orienteers. *Perceptual and Motor Skills* 62(2), 491-498. http://dx.doi.org/10.2466/pms.1986.62.2.491

p. 196 'Cricketers bowl less accurately'
Devlin, L., Fraser, S., Barras, N. & Hawley, J. (2001). Moderate levels of hypohydration impairs bowling accuracy but not bowling velocity in skilled cricket players. *Journal of Science and Medicine in Sport* 4(2), 179-187. http://dx.doi.org/10.1016/s1440-2440(01)80028-1

p. 196 'Tennis players' ground strokes'
Davey, P., Thorpe, R. & Williams, C. (2002). Fatigue decreases skilled tennis performance. *Journal of Sports Sciences* 20(4), 311-318. http://dx.doi.org/10.1080/026404102753576080

p. 197 'the Iowa Gambling Task'
The Iowa Gambling task is usually presented on a computer screen. Participants see four virtual decks of cards and are told that each time they choose a card they'll win some money. The aim of the game is to win as much money as possible. Occasionally, though, they'll pick a card that causes them to lose money. The four decks are either 'good' – they'll win the player money in the long run, or 'bad' – they'll lose the player money over time. In theory, players with normal risk-processing abilities should learn to pick the good decks more than the bad.

p. 200 'Stroop test'
The marshmallow test – often used with children – is another way of measuring response inhibition. Kids have to inhibit their desire to eat a marshmallow with the promise that they'll get an extra one if they don't eat it.

p. 200 'one fairly typical example was published in 2014'
Pageaux, B., Lepers, R., Dietz, K. & Marcora, S. (2014). Response inhibition impairs subsequent self-paced endurance performance. *European Journal of Applied Physiology* 114(5), 1095-1105. http://dx.doi.org/10.1007/s00421-014-2838-5

p. 201 'another group watched a documentary about the Orient Express'
Marcora, S., Staiano, W. & Manning, V. (2009). Mental fatigue impairs

physical performance in humans. *Journal of Applied Physiology* 106(3), 857-864. http://dx.doi.org/10.1152/japplphysiol.91324.2008

p. 201 'One of the most important studies in the field of exercise physiology'
Fletcher, W. & Hopkins, F. (1907). Lactic acid in amphibian muscle. *The Journal of Physiology* 35(4), 247-309. http://dx.doi.org/10.1113/jphysiol.1907.sp001194

p. 203 'When you start running'
Caesar, E.(2015). *Two Hours*. New York: Viking.

p. 203 'Mind is everything' – Paavo Nurmi
Noakes, T. (2012). Fatigue is a Brain-Derived Emotion that Regulates the Exercise Behavior to Ensure the Protection of Whole Body Homeostasis. *Frontiers in Physiology* 3. http://dx.doi.org/10.3389/fphys.2012.00082

p. 204 'According to legend'
Apparently there's a bit more to this story, as one of my friends who is more clued up on Greek legend than I am informs me. Pheidippides had done quite a lot of running before this point – to Sparta before Marathon – and had been selected for the task of delivering messages because he was Athens' best runner.

p. 204 'As I entered the stadium'
Burnton, S. (2012). 50 stunning Olympic moments No 16: Dorando Pietri's marathon, 1908. *Guardian*. Retrieved 29 November 2015, from http://www.theguardian.com/sport/2012/feb/29/50-stunning-olympic-moments

p. 207 'memorises how sections of road feel'
An interesting point on neural plasticity from Simon Wheatcroft: 'The one thing I've really noticed is how quick I can react to the feeling of something changing underfoot, because for example if I'm just walking, 'cause I've got small children and there's a toy – I can instantly change how much pressure I'm putting on my foot and switch to the other foot so I don't break the toy and just glide around, whereas a lot of people just step on the toy and break it. I'm at the point now where I can just move round, walk on toys – I think that does probably come from how much time I've dedicated to feeling what it's like underfoot.'

p. 208 'used EEG caps to measure the brains of cyclists'
Hilty, L., Langer, N., Pascual-Marqui, R., Boutellier, U. & Lutz, K. (2011). Fatigue-induced increase in intracortical communication between mid/anterior insular and motor cortex during cycling exercise. *European Journal of Neuroscience* 34(12), 2035-2042. http://dx.doi.org/10.1111/j.1460-9568.2011.07909.x

p. 208 'an ingenious contraption'
Fontes, E., Okano, A., De Guio, F., Schabort, E., Min, L. & Basset, F. et

al. (2013). Brain activity and perceived exertion during cycling exercise: an fMRI study. *British Journal of Sports Medicine* 49(8), 556-560. http://dx.doi.org/10.1136/bjsports-2012-091924

p. 209 'the way people are flung across the room when they get electric shocks' Epstein, D. (2014). Are athletes really getting faster, better, stronger? TED2014. Retrieved from: https://www.ted.com/talks/david_epstein_are_athletes_really_getting_faster_better_stronger?language=en

p. 212 'self-talk'

Eichner, E. (2015). Self-Talk, Deception, and Placebo Power in Sports Performance. *Current Sports Medicine Reports* 14(3), 147-148. http://dx.doi.org/10.1249/jsr.0000000000000153

p. 212 'Isner trained in Florida'

Caesar, E. (2011). The greatest Wimbledon match of all time. *GQ*. Retrieved 29 November 2015, from http://www.gq-magazine.co.uk/entertainment/articles/2011-06/03/gq-sport-wimbledon-nicolas-mahut-john-isner-tennis

p. 213 'Working with the Ministry of Defence'

McClusky, M. *Faster, Higher, Stronger.*

p. 215 'taste some milkshakes'

Crum, A., Corbin, W., Brownell, K. & Salovey, P. (2011). Mind over milkshakes: Mindsets, not just nutrients, determine ghrelin response. *Health Psychology* 30(4), 424-429. http://dx.doi.org/10.1037/a0023467

p. 215 'asked cyclists on exercise bikes'

Northumbria University. (17 October 2011). Pushing the limits of performance. ScienceDaily. Retrieved 29 November 2015, from www.sciencedaily.com/releases/2011/10/111017075514.htm

p. 216 'researchers can change the temperature and humidity'

Castle, P., Maxwell, N., Allchorn, A., Mauger, A. & White, D. (2011). Deception of ambient and body core temperature improves self paced cycling in hot, humid conditions. *European Journal of Applied Physiology* 112(1), 377-385. http://dx.doi.org/10.1007/s00421-011-1988-y

p. 218 'by smiling while running, for example – can improve your endurance'

Hutchinson, A. (2014). What Is Fatigue? *New Yorker*. Retrieved 29 November 2015, from http://www.newyorker.com/tech/elements/what-is-fatigue

Blanchfield, A., Hardy, J. & Marcora, S. (2014). Non-conscious visual cues related to affect and action alter perception of effort and endurance performance. *Frontiers in Human Neuroscience* 8. http://dx.doi.org/10.3389/fnhum.2014.00967

Another potential technology that might help is musical in nature. Researchers linked exercise machines in a gym to music-making kits which were synced to the pattern and force of the athletes' movements. The faster they lifted, the more intense the music and vice versa. They found that athletes who created their own music reported a lower perception of effort, produced more force and used less oxygen. Music streaming site Spotify has already developed an app that takes into account your heart rate when selecting tracks, so this kind of technology may be closer than you think.

Fritz, T., Hardikar, S., Demoucron, M., Niessen, M., Demey, M. & Giot, O. et al. (2013). Musical agency reduces perceived exertion during strenuous physical performance. *Proceedings of the National Academy of Sciences* 110(44), 17784-17789. http://dx.doi.org/10.1073/pnas.1217252110

p. 218 'Brain zapping'

Background from Santa Monica comes from a series of articles on RedBull.com: http://www.redbull.com/us/en/stories/1331658218665/red-bull-project-endurance

Also Alex Hutchinson article for *Outside*: http://www.outsideonline.com/1926551/your-body-brain-doping

p. 219 'gave 10 cyclists 20 minutes of tDCS'

Okano, A., Fontes, E., Montenegro, R., Farinatti, P., Cyrino, E. & Li, L. et al. (2013). Brain stimulation modulates the autonomic nervous system, rating of perceived exertion and performance during maximal exercise. *British Journal of Sports Medicine* 49(18), 1213-1218. http://dx.doi.org/10.1136/bjsports-2012-091658

p. 219 'tDCS of the motor cortex improved endurance'

Cogiamanian, F., Marceglia, S., Ardolino, G., Barbieri, S. & Priori, A. (2007). Improved isometric force endurance after transcranial direct current stimulation over the human motor cortical areas. *European Journal of Neuroscience* 26(1), 242-249. http://dx.doi.org/10.1111/j.1460-9568.2007.05633.x

p. 220 'Brain stimulation shouldn't be taken lightly'

Dana.org. Could Neurodoping Enhance Sporting Performance? Retrieved 29 November 2015, from http://dana.org/News/Details.aspx?id=43280

p. 221 'Strategies that modulate'

Globe and Mail. (2013). Don't blame your body if you tire out. Retrieved 29 November 2015, from http://www.theglobeandmail.com/life/health-and-fitness/dont-blame-your-body-if-you-tire-out/article11573542/

CHAPTER TEN

p. 230 'The pilot can generally see and hear'
Newman, D. (2014).*Flying Fast Jets.* Farnham, Surrey: Ashgate Publishing Ltd.

p. 232 'affect the way you perceive the positioning of your limbs'
Lackner, J. & DiZio, P. (1992). Gravitoinertial force level affects the appreciation of limb position during muscle vibration. *Brain Research* 592(1-2), 175-180. http://dx.doi.org/10.1016/0006-8993(92)91673-3

p. 232 'G-force makes it feel as though your body is being squeezed'
Norton, C. (2010). Formula One drivers feel the G-force. Telegraph.co.uk. Retrieved 29 November 2015, from http://www.telegraph.co.uk/motoring/motorsport/7681665/Formula-One-drivers-feel-the-G-force.html

CHAPTER ELEVEN

p. 234 'Sometimes I would recite poetry from the ring'
Nowinski, C. & Ventura, J. *Head Games.*

p. 237 'A survey of players in the Canadian Football League'
Delaney, J., Lacroix, V., Leclerc, S. & Johnston, K. (2002). Concussions Among University Football and Soccer Players. *Clinical Journal of Sport Medicine* 12(6), 331-338. http://dx.doi.org/10.1097/00042752-200211000-00003

p. 237 'Two studies into high schoolers'
Langburt, W., Cohen, B., Akhthar, N., O'Neill, K. & Lee, J. (2001). Incidence of Concussion in High School Football Players of Ohio and Pennsylvania. *Journal of Child Neurology* 16(02), 083. http://dx.doi.org/10.2310/7010.2001.6943

McCrea, M., Hammeke, T., Olsen, G., Leo, P. & Guskiewicz, K. (2004). Unreported Concussion in High School Football Players. *Clinical Journal of Sport Medicine* 14(1), 13-17. http://dx.doi.org/10.1097/00042752-200401000-00003

p. 241 'Please see that my brain is given to the NFL's brain bank' – Dave Duerson
A fuller extract from the Duerson note: 'My mind slips. Thoughts get crossed. Cannot find my words. Major growth on the back of skull on lower left side. Feel really alone. Thinking of other NFL players with brain injuries. Sometimes, simple spelling becomes a chore, and my eyesite goes blurry ... I think something is seriously damaged in my brain, too. I cannot tell you how many times I saw stars in games, but I

know there were many times that I would "wake up" well after a game, and we were all at dinner.'

p. 241 'the autopsy table of Dr Bennet Omalu'
Omalu was played by Will Smith in the movie *Concussion*, which was released in the UK in February 2016. It's based on a 2009 *GQ* article: http://www.gq.com/story/nfl-players-brain-dementia-study-memory-concussions

p. 243 'enough to fill another book'
If you're looking for one, try: *League of Denial: The NFL, Concussions and the Battle for Truth* (New York: Crown Archetype, 2013).

p. 250 'Players can view the baseline test as an obstacle in their way for getting back playing'
ESPN Scrum.com. 'Players are deliberately cheating concussion tests'. Retrieved 29 November 2015, from http://en.espn.co.uk/scrum/rugby/story/208943.html

p. 253 'Death by industrial disease'
Katwala, A. (2014). *Death by Industrial Disease. Sport* magazine 399.

p. 253 'You find it so hard to believe that football can do that'
Sky Sports. Jeff Astle's family unhappy with authorities following research over his death. Retrieved 29 November 2015, from http://www.skysports.com/football/news/11698/9333913/jeff-astles-family-unhappy-with-authorities-following-research-over-his-death

p. 253 'World Cup-winning captain Bellini'
Knight, S. (2014). The cost of the header. *New Yorker*. http://www.newyorker.com/news/sporting-scene/cost-header

p. 254 'Michael Lipton and colleagues'
Radiology: Soccer Heading Is Associated with White Matter Microstructural and Cognitive Abnormalities. (2013). *Radiology*. Retrieved from http://pubs.rsna.org/doi/full/10.1148/radiol.13130545

p. 255 'followed two high school women's football teams'
Poole, V., Breedlove, E., Shenk, T., Abbas, K., Robinson, M. & Leverenz, L. et al. (2015). Sub-Concussive Hit Characteristics Predict Deviant Brain Metabolism in Football Athletes. *Developmental Neuropsychology* 40(1), 12-17. http://dx.doi.org/10.1080/87565641.2014.984810

p. 255 'The percentage of 100 g hits'
Ingle, S. (2015). Research reveals footballers are still heading for serious trouble. *Guardian*. Retrieved 29 November 2015, from http://www.theguardian.com/football/blog/2015/nov/01/football-heading-brain-damage

p. 257 'Traditional helmet technology in the NFL'
Rowson, S., Duma, S., Greenwald, R., Beckwith, J., Chu, J. & Guskiewicz,

K. et al. (2014). Can helmet design reduce the risk of concussion in football? *Journal of Neurosurgery* 120(4), 919-922. http://dx.doi.org/10.3171/2014.1.jns13916

p. 259 'A gene called ApoE4'

Gavett, B., Stern, R. & McKee, A. (2011). Chronic Traumatic Encephalopathy: A Potential Late Effect of Sport-Related Concussive and Subconcussive Head Trauma. *Clinics in Sports Medicine* 30(1), 179-188. http://dx.doi.org/10.1016/j.csm.2010.09.007

p. 260 'It binds with any tau in the brain'

UCLA Newsroom.UCLA study finds characteristic pattern of protein deposits in brains of retired NFL players who suffered concussions. Retrieved 29 November 2015, from http://newsroom.ucla.edu/releases/ucla-study-finds-characteristic-pattern-of-protein-deposits-in-brains-of-retired-nfl-players-who-suffered-concussions

USA TODAY. (2013). Study gives hope for brain disease treatment. Retrieved 29 November 2015, from http://www.usatoday.com/story/sports/nfl/2013/01/22/nfl-concussions-cte-junior-seau/1855555/

p. 261 'estrone, one of the body's three naturally occurring oestrogen hormones'

ANI News. Estrogen hormone 'may have protective ability after traumatic brain injury'. Retrieved 29 November 2015, from http://www.aninews.in/newsdetail9/story47429/estrogen-hormone-039-may-have-protective-ability-after-traumatic-brain-injury-039-.html

p. 261 'light therapy'

Naeser, M., Saltmarche, A., Krengel, M., Hamblin, M. & Knight, J. (2011). Improved Cognitive Function After Transcranial, Light-Emitting Diode Treatments in Chronic, Traumatic Brain Injury: Two Case Reports. *Photomedicine and Laser Surgery* 29(5), 351-358. http://dx.doi.org/10.1089/pho.2010.2814

CHAPTER 12

p. 271 'a harrowing watch'

https://www.youtube.com/watch?v=-OBX25ix4eU

p. 272 'Someone who takes risks to accomplish something'

Ngm.nationalgeographic.com. (2013). The Mystery of Risk. Retrieved 29 November 2015, from http://ngm.nationalgeographic.com/2013/06/125-risk-takers/gwin-text

p. 272 'used fMRI to measure blood flow'

Wittmann, B., Daw, N., Seymour, B. & Dolan, R. (2008). Striatal Activity

Underlies Novelty-Based Choice in Humans. *Neuron* 58(6), 967-973. http://dx.doi.org/10.1016/j.neuron.2008.04.027

p. 272 'We think this piece, the VS, adds zing – a reward when we encounter novel things'
Outside Online. (2009). This Is Your Brain on Adventure. Retrieved 29 November 2015, from http://www.outsideonline.com/1896581/your-brain-adventure

p. 273 'Sensation Seeking Scale'
Try it out for yourself here: http://www.bbc.co.uk/science/humanbody/mind/surveys/sensation/index_1.shtml?age=&gender=&occupation=&education=

p. 273 'I tried to get him into his car'
People.com. Heroes Among Us. Retrieved 29 November 2015, from http://www.people.com/people/archive/article/0,,20129834,00.html

p. 273 'These people are motivated by risk, uncertainty, novelty, variety'
Partners.nytimes.com. (1998). The Thrill of Risk, and Other Reasons Why. Retrieved 29 November 2015, from https://partners.nytimes.com/library/sports/outdoors/031198adventure-risk.html

p. 274 'similarities between drug addicts in rehab and high-risk sport participants'
Franques, P. (2003). Sensation seeking as a common factor in opioid dependent subjects and high risk sport practicing subjects. A cross sectional study. *Drug and Alcohol Dependence* 69(2), 121-126. http://dx.doi.org/10.1016/s0376-8716(02)00309-5

p. 275 'studied two different groups of soldiers'
Morgan, C., Wang, S., Southwick, S., Rasmusson, A., Hazlett, G., Hauger, R. & Charney, D. (2000). Plasma neuropeptide-Y concentrations in humans exposed to military survival training. *Biological Psychiatry* 47(10), 902-909. http://dx.doi.org/10.1016/s0006-3223(99)00239-5

p. 276 'The more someone struggles'
Newsweek.com. Retrieved 29 November 2015, from http://www.newsweek.com/ultimate-stress-test-special-forces-training-82749

p. 278 'Every time I step off the edge I'm scared'
Winter Sessions – The Reality of Falling with Ted Davenport: https://www.youtube.com/watch?v=JTFp44Ib4Cc

CHAPTER THIRTEEN

p. 280 'a head-spinning combination of a cattle market and a speed-dating session'

Reynolds, N. (2010). American football meets speed dating. bbc.co.uk. Retrieved 29 November 2015, from http://www.bbc.co.uk/blogs/neilreynolds/2010/02/nfl_combine_marks_the_start_of.html

p. 281 'the unofficial average score for a quarterback'
Lehrer, J. (2011). True Grit. *ESPN* (18 April 2011 edn). Retrieved from http://espn.go.com/nfl/draft2011/news/story?id=6299428

p. 281 'A study by economists David Berri and Rob Simmons'
Berri, D. & Simmons, R. (2009). Catching a draft: on the process of selecting quarterbacks in the National Football League amateur draft. *Journal of Productivity Analysis* 35(1), 37-49. http://dx.doi.org/10.1007/s11123-009-0154-6

p. 283 'One study of ice hockey players'
Furley, P. & Memmert, D. (2012). Working memory capacity as controlled attention in tactical decision making. *Journal of Sport & Exercise Psychology* 34 (3), 322–344 10.1371/journal.pone.0062278

p. 283 'tested a group of people on their overall baseball knowledge'
Hambrick, D. & Engle, R. (2002). Effects of Domain Knowledge, Working Memory Capacity, and Age on Cognitive Performance: An Investigation of the Knowledge-Is-Power Hypothesis. *Cognitive Psychology* 44(4), 339-387. http://dx.doi.org/10.1006/cogp.2001.0769

p. 283 'A group of 57 pianists'
Meinz, E. J. & Hambrick, D.Z. (2010). Deliberate practice is necessary but not sufficient to explain individual differences in piano sight-reading skill: the role of working memory capacity. *Psychological Science* 21(7), 914-919.

p. 284 'an hour a day, between three and five days a week for a year'
Ericsson, K. A. et al. (1980). Acquisition of a memory skill. *Science* 208, 1181–1182.

p. 284 'perform better on measures of processing speed, attention and executive function'
Voss, M., Kramer, A., Basak, C., Prakash, R. & Roberts, B. (2009). Are expert athletes expert in the cognitive laboratory? A meta-analytic review of cognition and sport expertise. *Applied Cognitive Psychology* 24(6), 812-826. http://dx.doi.org/10.1002/acp.1588

p. 285 'In one study of executive function'
Chaddock, L., Neider, M., Voss, M., Gaspar, J. & Kramer, A. (2011). Do Athletes Excel At Everyday Tasks?.*Medicine & Science in Sports & Exercise* 1. http://dx.doi.org/10.1249/mss.0b013e318218ca74

p. 285 'One study of Swedish footballers'
Verburgh, L., Scherder, E., van Lange, P. & Oosterlaan, J. (2014).

Executive Functioning in Highly Talented Soccer Players. *PLoS ONE* 9(3), e91254. http://dx.doi.org/10.1371/journal.pone.0091254

p. 287 'There's not going to be a single gene that determines success or failure'
Mail Online. (2014). Two Premier League clubs sign up with top genetic profiling company. Retrieved 29 November 2015, from http://www.dailymail.co.uk/sport/football/article-2582714/Two-Premier-League-clubs-sign-genetics-company-learn-DNA-profiles-players.html

p. 287 'We're just hoping to reduce the risk'
This echoes what's happening for concussion and CTE with screening for the ApoE4 gene.

p. 288 'One version of a gene called COMT has been linked with improved performance in working memory tasks'
Dumontheil, I., Roggeman, C., Ziermans, T., Peyrard-Janvid, M., Matsson, H., Kere, J. & Klingberg, T. (2011). Influence of the COMT Genotype on Working Memory and Brain Activity Changes During Development. *Biological Psychiatry* 70(3), 222-229. http://dx.doi.org/10.1016/j.biopsych.2011.02.027
Wardle, M., de Wit, H., Penton-Voak, I., Lewis, G. & Munafò, M. (2013). Lack of Association Between COMT and Working Memory in a Population-Based Cohort of Healthy Young Adults. *Neuropsychopharmacology* 38(7), 1253-1263. http://dx.doi.org/10.1038/npp.2013.24

p. 288 'linked to processing speed'
Ibrahim-Verbaas, C., Bressler, J., Debette, S., Schuur, M., Smith, A. & Bis, J. et al. (2015). GWAS for executive function and processing speed suggests involvement of the CADM2 gene. *Molecular Psychiatry*. http://dx.doi.org/10.1038/mp.2015.37

p. 288 'differences in executive function are almost entirely genetic'
Individual differences in executive function are almost entirely inherited, according to one twin study which tested three aspects of it and concluded that genes account for 99 per cent of the difference.
Friedman, N., Miyake, A., Young, S., DeFries, J., Corley, R. & Hewitt, J. (2008). Individual differences in executive functions are almost entirely genetic in origin. *Journal of Experimental Psychology: General* 137(2), 201-225. http://dx.doi.org/10.1037/0096-3445.137.2.201

p. 289 'Dr Claude Bouchard tested'
This study, and others from the HERITAGE family study, are described in *The Sports Gene*.

p. 290 'About 65 per cent of people have the Val66Val version'
Baj, G., Carlino, D., Gardossi, L. & Tongiorgi, E. (2013). Toward a

unified biological hypothesis for the BDNF Val66Met-associated memory deficits in humans: a model of impaired dendritic mRNA trafficking. *Frontiers in Neuroscience* 7, 188. http://dx.doi.org/10.3389/fnins.2013.00188

Kleim, J., Chan, S., Pringle, E., Schallert, K., Procaccio, V., Jimenez, R. & Cramer, S. (2006). BDNF val66met polymorphism is associated with modified experience-dependent plasticity in human motor cortex. *Nature Neuroscience* 9(6), 735-737. http://dx.doi.org/10.1038/nn1699

Cheeran, B., Talelli, P., Mori, F., Koch, G., Suppa, A. & Edwards, M. et al. (2008). A common polymorphism in the brain-derived neurotrophic factor gene (BDNF) modulates human cortical plasticity and the response to rTMS. *The Journal of Physiology* 586(23), 5717-5725. http://dx.doi.org/10.1113/jphysiol.2008.159905

p. 291 'Grit is passion and perseverance for very long-term goals'

Duckworth, A. L. (2013). The key to success? Grit. TED Talks Education. https://www.ted.com/talks/angela_lee_duckworth_the_key_to_success_grit?language=en

Try this online version of the grit test: https://sasupenn.qualtrics.com/jfe/form/SV_06f6QSOS2pZW9qR

Or this printable 12-item scale: https://www.sas.upenn.edu/~duckwort/images/12-item%20Grit%20Scale.05312011.pdf

p. 292 'Duckworth tested contestants at the National Spelling Bee'

Duckworth, A., Kirby, T., Tsukayama, E., Berstein, H. & Ericsson, K. (2010). Deliberate Practice Spells Success: Why Grittier Competitors Triumph at the National Spelling Bee. *Social Psychological and Personality Science* 2(2), 174-181. http://dx.doi.org/10.1177/1948550610385872

p. 293 'one that used accelerometers'

Fisher, A., van Jaarsveld, C., Llewellyn, C. & Wardle, J. (2010). Environmental Influences on Children's Physical Activity: Quantitative Estimates Using a Twin Design. *PLoS ONE* 5(4), e10110. http://dx.doi.org/10.1371/journal.pone.0010110

p. 293 'more than 37,000 pairs of twins'

Stubbe, J. H., Boomsma, D.I., Vink, J. M., Cornes, B. K. & Martin, N. G. et al. (2006). Genetic influences on exercise participation in 37,051 twin pairs from seven countries. *PLoS ONE* 1, e22. [PMC free article] [PubMed]

p. 293 'he bred mice that were born to run'

Rhodes, J. S., Cammie, S. C. & Garland, T. Jr. (2005). Neurobiology of Mice Selected for High Voluntary Wheel-Running Activity. *Integrative and Comparative Biology* 45(3), 438-55.

p. 294 'the couch potato gene'
Zhang, Z., Hao, C., Li, C., Zang, D., Zhao, J. & Li, X. et al. (2014). Mutation of SLC35D3 Causes Metabolic Syndrome by Impairing Dopamine Signaling in Striatal D1 Neurons. *PLoS Genetics* 10(2), e1004124. http://dx.doi.org/10.1371/journal.pgen.1004124

p. 294 'Science says grit comes from both nature and nurture'
Tam, R. (2013). MacArthur fellow Angela Duckworth: Test kids' grit, not just their IQ. *Washington Post.* Retrieved 30 November 2015, from https://www.washingtonpost.com/blogs/she-the-people/wp/2013/09/27/macarthur-fellow-angela-duckworth-test-kids-grit-not-just-their-iq/

p. 296 'may inherit that adaptability'
Gapp, K., Soldado-Magraner, S., Alvarez-Sánchez, M., Bohacek, J., Vernaz, G. & Shu, H. et al. (2014). Early life stress in fathers improves behavioural flexibility in their offspring. *Nature Communications* 5, 5466. http://dx.doi.org/10.1038/ncomms6466

p. 296 'an EEG experiment at Michigan State University'
Moser, J., Schroder, H., Heeter, C., Moran, T. & Lee, Y. (2011). Mind Your Errors: Evidence for a Neural Mechanism Linking Growth Mind-Set to Adaptive Posterror Adjustments. *Psychological Science* 22(12), 1484-1489. http://dx.doi.org/10.1177/0956797611419520

p. 297 'the brain sits up and pays attention when things go wrong'
Syed, M. (2015). *Black Box Thinking.* London: Hodder & Stoughton.

CHAPTER FOURTEEN

p. 299 'Moldova approached me first'
Maul, R. (2015). Aaron Cook: I switched to Moldova as national anthem means NOTHING to me. Express.co.uk. Retrieved 30 November 2015, from http://www.express.co.uk/sport/othersport/584915/Aaron-Cook-Taekwondo-Moldova-Switch-English-National-Anthem

INDEX